Emergency Nurse Practitioner
Scope and Standards of Practice

Wesley D. Davis, DNP, ENP-C, FNP-C, AGACNP-BC, CEN, FAANP, FAEN, is an emergency nurse practitioner (ENP) with over 2 decades of clinical experience in emergency care. Dr. Davis developed a dual family and ENP program at the University of South Alabama, where he currently serves as an associate professor and the program coordinator. As a practicing clinician, Dr. Davis is an emergency and acute care nurse practitioner at Crook County Medical Services District, a critical access hospital in Wyoming.

Dr. Davis obtained his bachelor of science in nursing at the Chamberlain College of Nursing and both his master of science in nursing and his doctor of nursing practice at the University of South Alabama. His service includes being president of the American Academy of Emergency Nurse Practitioners (AAENP), a past president of the Wyoming Council of Advanced Practice Nurses, and associate editor of the *Advanced Emergency Nursing Journal*.

Dr. Davis spearheaded and led a multi-organizational collaborative initiative to align two sets of ENP competencies into a single version, as presented in this book.

Dr. Davis is widely recognized for his contributions to the ENP profession through numerous professional awards, including a Fellow of the Academy of Emergency Nursing, the University of South Alabama College of Nursing Alumni Society Emerging Alumni Award, the Emergency Nurses Association Frank L. Cole Nurse Practitioner Award, and a Fellow of the American Association of Nurse Practitioners (AANP).

Dian Dowling Evans, PhD, FNP-BC, ENP-C, FAAN, FAANP, is professor emeritus and former program director of the Nell Hodgson Woodruff School of Nursing at Emory University. With over 30 years of clinical experience as an ENP, Dr. Evans helped to pioneer and advance the ENP role. Her contributions include collaborating with a core group of ENP national leaders to establish the AAENP, serving as a founding board member and past chair. During her tenure, she established and led the ENP Special Practice Group for the AANP and the ENP Special Interest Group for the National Organization of Nurse Practitioner Faculties.

Recognized as a leader within the ENP profession, Dr. Evans is actively involved in national ENP policy initiatives, certification exam development, and curricular standards. She currently serves as the Research to Practice column editor for the *Advanced Emergency Nursing Journal* and has extensive publications and national and international presentations on emergency medicine topics, the ENP role, and ENP education. Dr. Evans's efforts and contributions to the nursing profession have been recognized through induction into the Fellows of the AANP and the American Academy of Nursing.

ABOUT THE AMERICAN ACADEMY OF EMERGENCY NURSE PRACTITIONERS

The AAENP was founded in 2014 in response to the growing need for standardized ENP education and competency validation for the estimated 14,600 nurse practitioners (NPs) practicing in emergency care. In 2019, approximately 7.5% of NPs reported working in an emergency care setting (AANP, 2019). As of 2022, there are more than 355,000 NPs in the United States (AANP, 2022). As the professional organization for ENPs, the AAENP now represents nearly 27,000 NPs working in emergency care settings and over 1,700 board-certified ENPs (D. Tyler, personal communication, April 15, 2023). Together with strategic partner organizations and policy makers, the AAENP has established itself as a leader in emergency care.

MISSION STATEMENT

The AAENP promotes high-quality, evidence-based practice for nurse practitioners providing emergency care for patients of all ages and acuities in collaboration with an interdisciplinary team. More specifically, the academy seeks to

- Establish guidelines for quality and safety in emergency healthcare.
- Encourage continuing clinical education of emergency nurse practitioners.
- Support training and education in emergency care.
- Facilitate research in emergency care.
- Collaborate with professional health organizations and academic institutions.

VISION

The AAENP is the preeminent professional organization serving as the expert and unified voice for nurse practitioners in emergency care.

REFERENCES

American Association of Nurse Practitioners. (2019). *Nurse practitioner compensation*. https://storage.aanp.org/www/documents/no-index/research/2019-NP-Sample-Survey-Report.pdf.
American Association of Nurse Practitioners. (2022). *NP fact sheet*. https://storage.aanp.org/www/documents/NPFacts__111022.pdf.

Emergency Nurse Practitioner Scope and Standards of Practice

Wesley D. Davis, DNP, ENP-C, FNP-C, AGACNP-BC, CEN, FAANP, FAEN

Dian Dowling Evans, PhD, FNP-BC, ENP-C, FAAN, FAANP

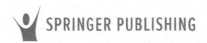 SPRINGER PUBLISHING

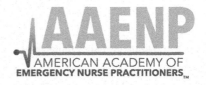 AMERICAN ACADEMY OF EMERGENCY NURSE PRACTITIONERS™

Springer Publishing Company, LLC
www.springerpub.com
connect.springerpub.com

Acquisitions Editor: John Zaphyr
Production Editor: Diana Osborne
Compositor: Diacritech

ISBN: 978-0-8261-7847-3
ebook ISBN: 978-0-8261-7848-0
DOI: 10.1891/9780826178480

SUPPLEMENT:
ENP Program Evaluation Form ISBN: 978-0-8261-7849-7

23 24 25 26 / 5 4 3 2 1

The author and the publisher of this Work have made every effort to use sources believed to be reliable to provide information that is accurate and compatible with the standards generally accepted at the time of publication. Because medical science is continually advancing, our knowledge base continues to expand. Therefore, as new information becomes available, changes in procedures become necessary. We recommend that the reader always consult current research and specific institutional policies before performing any clinical procedure or delivering any medication. The author and publisher shall not be liable for any special, consequential, or exemplary damages resulting, in whole or in part, from the readers' use of, or reliance on, the information contained in this book. The publisher has no responsibility for the persistence or accuracy of URLs for external or third-party Internet websites referred to in this publication and does not guarantee that any content on such websites is, or will remain, accurate or appropriate.

Library of Congress Cataloging-in-Publication Data

Names: Davis, Wesley D., editor. | Evans, Dian Dowling, editor. | American Academy of Emergency Nurse
   Practitioners, issuing body.
Title: Emergency nurse practitioner scope and standards of practice / [edited by] Wesley D Davis,
   Dian Dowling Evans.
Description: [Scottsdale, Ariz.] : AAENP, American Academy of Emergency Nurse Practitioners; New York :
   Springer Publishing, [2024] | Includes bibliographical references and index. | Summary: "Since the
   emergency medicine specialty's inception in the 1960s, APRNs have worked alongside physician colleagues
   providing emergency care to patients of all ages and acuities. As emergency care evolved and ED census
   levels rapidly grew during the 1990s, utilization of APRNs was essential to increasing emergency staffing,
   efficiency, patient satisfaction, and quality of care. The growing need for APRNs prepared with emergency-
   specific competencies resulted in the creation of the emergency nurse practitioner (ENP) profession and the
   establishment of educational and training programs to support the role"– Provided by publisher.
Identifiers: LCCN 2023045458 (print) | LCCN 2023045459 (ebook) | ISBN 9780826178473 (paperback) |
   ISBN 9780826178480 (ebook)
Subjects: MESH: Emergency Nursing–standards | Nurse Practitioners–standards | Clinical Competence |
   Nurse's Role | Emergencies–nursing | United States
Classification: LCC RC86.7 (print) | LCC RC86.7 (ebook) | NLM WY 152.4 | DDC 616.02/5–dc23/eng/20231030
LC record available at https://lccn.loc.gov/2023045458
LC ebook record available at https://lccn.loc.gov/2023045459

Contact sales@springerpub.com to receive discount rates on bulk purchases.

Publisher's Note: **New and used products purchased from third-party sellers are not guaranteed for quality, authenticity, or access to any included digital components.**

Printed in the United States of America by Gasch Printing.

CONTENTS

CONTRIBUTORS

Amanda Comer, DNP, APRN, FNP-BC, ACNP-BC, ENP-BC, ENP-C, System Director, Advanced Practice Providers, Baptist Memorial Health Care Corporation, Memphis, Tennessee

Wesley D. Davis, DNP, ENP-C, FNP-C, AGACNP-BC, CEN, FAANP, FAEN, President, American Academy of Emergency Nurse Practitioners, Associate Professor, Dual FNP/Emergency Nurse Practitioner Coordinator, University of South Alabama College of Nursing, Mobile, Alabama

Dian Dowling Evans, PhD, FNP-BC, ENP-C, FAAN, FAANP, Professor Emeritus, Clinical Track & Family/Emergency Nurse Practitioner, Nell Hodgson Woodruff School of Nursing, Emory University, Atlanta, Georgia

Valerie Fuller, PhD, DNP, AGACNP-BC, FNP-BC, FNAP, FAANP, Board President and APRN member of the Maine State Board of Nursing, Nurse Practitioner, Department of Surgery, Maine Medical Center, Portland, Maine; Assistant Professor of Surgery, Tufts University School of Medicine, Boston, Massachusetts

Bradley Goettl, DNP, APRN, FNP-C, AGACNP-BC, ENP-C, FAANP, FAEN, FAAN, Assistant Director, Office of Advanced Practice Providers, Program Director, APP Fellowships, UT Southwestern Medical Center, Dallas, Texas

Chivas Guillote, DNP, APRN, ENP-C, FNP-C, AGACNP-BC, LP, Vice President of Clinical Services, Harris County Emergency Corps, Houston, Texas

Melanie Gibbons Hallman, DNP, CRNP, FNP-BC, ACNP-BC, ENP-C, CNS, FAEN, FAAN, Associate Professor, Emergency Nurse Practitioner Subspeciality Pathway Co-Coordinator, The University of Alabama at Birmingham School of Nursing, Birmingham, Alabama

David House, DNP, CRNP, ENP-C, FNP-BC, CNS, CNE, CEN, FAEN, FAANP, Associate Professor, Emergency Nurse Practitioner Subspeciality Pathway Co-Coordinator, The University of Alabama at Birmingham School of Nursing, Birmingham, Alabama

K. Sue Hoyt, PhD, RN, FNP-BC, ENP-C, FAEN, FAANP, FAAN, Professor, Hahn School of Nursing and Health Science, Beyster Institute for Nursing Research, Advanced Practice, and Simulation, University of San Diego, San Diego, California; EmergeED Consultation, San Diego, California; Editor-in-Chief, *Advanced Emergency Nursing Journal*, Wolters Kluwer/Lippincott, Williams & Wilkins

April Kapu, DNP, APRN, ACNP-BC, FAANP, FCCM, FAAN, Associate Dean Clinical and Community Partnerships, Vanderbilt University School of Nursing, Nashville, Tennessee

Lorna Schuman, PhD, FNP-C, ENP-C, ACNP-BC, ACNS-BC, FAAN, FAANP, Chair, American Academy of Nurse Practitioner Certification Board, Austin, Texas

Diane Tyler, PhD, RN, FNP-C, FNP-BC, CAE, FAANP, FAAN, Chief Executive Officer, American Academy of Nurse Practitioners Certification Board, Austin, Texas

Jennifer Wilbeck, DNP, ACNP-BC, ENP-C, FNP-C, FAAN, FAANP, Professor and Emergency NP Academic Director, Vanderbilt University School of Nursing, Nashville, Tennessee

EMERGENCY NURSE PRACTITIONER COMPETENCIES WORK GROUP

The 2021 emergency nurse practitioner competencies in this book represent the integration of previously published competencies from the American Academy of Emergency Nurse Practitioners (AAENP, 2018) and the Emergency Nurses Association (ENA, 2019). Members of the ENP Competencies Work Group include representatives from both the AAENP and the ENA. The following individuals comprised the group, which worked to synthesize and collate both sets of prior documents into a unified presentation of current emergency nurse practitioner competencies.

Wesley D. Davis, DNP, ENP-C, FNP-C, AGACNP-BC, CEN, FAANP, FAEN, Work Group Chairperson
University of South Alabama, Mobile, Alabama

Nancy Denke, DNP, ACNP-BC, FNP-BC, FAEN, CEN, CCRN
Arizona State University, Arizona

Melanie Gibbons Hallman, DNP, CRNP, FNP-BC, ACNP-BC, ENP-C, CNS, FAEN, FAAN, Work Group Chairperson
University of Alabama at Birmingham, Birmingham, Alabama

David House, DNP, FNP-BC, ENP-C, CNE, CNS, CEN, FAEN, FAANP
University of Alabama at Birmingham, Birmingham, Alabama

Diane Fuller Switzer, DNP, FNP-BC, ENP-C, ENP-BC, CCRN, CEN, FAEN, FAANP
Seattle University, Seattle, Washington

Jennifer Wilbeck, DNP, ACNP-BC, FNP-BC, ENP-C, FAANP, FAAN
Vanderbilt University, Nashville, Tennessee

EMERGENCY NURSE PRACTITIONER SCOPE AND STANDARDS WORK GROUP

The *Scope and Standards for Emergency Nurse Practitioner Practice* (2016) in this book represent the first official scope and standards for emergency nurse practitioners (ENPs). Subsequent guidelines for ENP education, certification, and practice are based on these scopes and standards. By establishing clear expectations for ENP practice and setting standards for education and certification, the scope and standards provide a strong foundation for the ongoing development of the role.

Dian Dowling Evans, PhD, FNP-BC, ENP-BC, FAAN, FAANP, Work Group Chairperson

AMERICAN ACADEMY OF EMERGENCY NURSE PRACTITIONER VALIDATION COMMITTEE

Wesley D. Davis, DNP, ENP-C, FNP-C, AGACNP-BC, CEN, FAANP, FAEN, Committee Chair

PREFACE

Since the emergency medicine specialty's inception in the 1960s, APRNs have worked alongside physician colleagues, providing emergency care to patients of all ages and acuities. As emergency care evolved and ED census levels rapidly grew during the 1990s, utilization of APRNs was essential to increasing emergency staffing, efficiency, patient satisfaction, and quality of care. The growing need for APRNs prepared with emergency-specific competencies resulted in the creation of the emergency nurse practitioner (ENP) profession and the establishment of educational and training programs to support the role.

Although several emergency-specific programs were offered to APRNs during the 1980s, the need for formalized emergency curricula grew significantly during the 1990s, fueled by the dramatic increases in ED census rates, the nationwide lack of access to primary care, and persistent emergency medicine workforce gaps. Momentum supporting the ENP role and profession accelerated with the publication of the *Consensus Model for APRN Regulation* that provided recommendations for licensure, accreditation, certification, and education of specialty prepared APRNs. Also, in 2008, the ENP core competencies were published by the Emergency Nurses Association (ENA), endorsed by the National Organization of Nurse Practitioner Faculties (NONPF). Finally, with recognition of the ENP specialty role by the National Council of State Boards of Nursing in 2010 and designation of emergency nursing as a specialty by the American Nurses Association in 2011, the ENP profession was officially established.

Over the past 35 years, ENP leaders, educators, researchers, and clinicians have diligently worked to further define the ENP role and educational preparation based on knowledge of changing practice trends and on scientifically derived national emergency medicine census data, including from the American College of Emergency Physicians' Benchmarking Alliance and the Centers for Disease Control and Prevention's National Hospital and Ambulatory Care Survey. Further efforts by ENP leaders led to the establishment in 2014 of the American Academy of Emergency Nurse Practitioners (AAENP), an organization solely dedicated to the ENP profession. Shortly thereafter, the AAENP collaborated with the American Academy of Nurse Practitioners Certification Board to conduct a large-scale role delineation study, leading to the development of a rigorous, psychometrically sound, nationally accredited ENP certification examination that launched in 2017. Over the next several years, the AAENP joined with the American Association of Nurse Practitioners (AANP) to establish the ENP Specialty Practice Group, providing a forum for ENPs from across the country to dialogue about practice and regulatory issues. Next, the AAENP established an ENP Special Interest Group with NONPF to provide ENP faculty with resources for ENP educational strategies. In 2021, leaders from the AAENP and the ENA joined to publish the revised ENP competencies which incorporated new practice trends and updated role delineation study findings. In addition to these accomplishments, ENP leaders have published extensively in peer-reviewed journals and presented nationally and internationally in support of the profession.

Emergency Nurse Practitioner Scope and Standards is dedicated to ENPs, educators, students, researchers, policy makers, employers, and to our physician and advanced practice colleagues to clarify the ENP role and its evidence-based foundation. This text contains the contributions of diverse national nursing leaders and dedicated ENPs who have worked tirelessly at the national, global, and local levels to advance the profession to ensure that ENPs are competent in delivering safe, accessible, high-quality, emergency care.

Emergency Nurse Practitioner Scope and Standards **offers an additional resource, ENP Program Evaluation Form, in PDF format with fill-in fields, which is accessible as a free chapter via the Table of Contents at https://connect.springerpub.com/content/book/978-0-8261-7848-0.**

Dian Dowling Evans, PhD, FNP-BC, ENP-C, FAAN, FAANP
Emeritus Professor, Emergency Nurse Practitioner Program, Nell Hodgson
Woodruff School of Nursing, Emory University, Atlanta, GA
Founding Board Member and Past Chair, American
Academy of Emergency Nurse Practitioners

ACKNOWLEDGMENTS

It is with great admiration and respect that we dedicate this book to Dr. Karen "Sue" Hoyt. As a true pioneer in the field of emergency nursing, Dr. Hoyt's contributions have been nothing short of transformative. Her unwavering dedication to advancing the emergency nurse practitioner role has left an indelible mark on our profession. We are grateful for her leadership and vision and for the countless ways she has inspired us all.

It is with great pleasure and gratitude that we dedicate this book to Dr. Elda Ramirez. As the founder of the American Academy of Emergency Nurse Practitioners, Dr. Ramirez has been a trailblazer in this field, leading the way for many nurse practitioners to provide the highest level of emergency care to those in need. Her vision and dedication have been an inspiration to us all, and this book serves as a testament to her enduring legacy.

Wesley D. Davis, DNP, ENP-C, FNP-C, AGACNP-BC, CEN, FAANP, FAEN

Dian Dowling Evans, PhD, FNP-BC, ENP-C, FAAN, FAANP

CHAPTER 1.1

Introduction

Wesley D. Davis

Scope and standards of practice are important components of professional practice. These concepts set out the scope of the emergency nurse practitioner's (ENP) job responsibilities and identify the acceptable behaviors that must be maintained to ensure quality and safe emergency care. Scope outlines the range of services, interventions, and assessments the ENP can perform. On the other hand, standards of practice are set rules and ethical principles that provide direction on how practice should be carried out and establish accountability expectations. Since ENPs provide care across the life span to all ages, care for a wide range of conditions from nonurgent to life threatening, and cover an in-depth knowledge base from obstetrics to orthopedics, a broad scope of practice is essential. When adhered to, the scope and standards of practice help to ensure that quality and safe care is consistently delivered by the ENP. The standards and competencies presented in this text are periodically reviewed to adapt to the evolving field of emergency care.

CHAPTER 2.1

Definition of Emergency Care

Wesley D. Davis

INTRODUCTION

A formal definition of emergency care is essential for regulatory bodies, such as boards of nursing, to establish practice guidelines and regulatory policies. Additionally, an evidence-based definition further guides the formation of academic programs, curricular standards, and performance assessments. The definition of emergency care is also useful to credentialing bodies, for provider privileging, and to insurers and payors. Through a concept analysis, an empirically defensible definition of emergency care was elucidated from the professional literature (Davis et al., 2020).

DEFINITION OF EMERGENCY CARE

> Emergency care occurs after a precipitating event, with recognition that medical help is required, having an element of severity or perceived severity, and providing access to emergency care treatment/services. Emergency care itself is the immediate evaluation and treatment of individuals with unexpected illness or injury with a perception of severity, with variance from minor to life-threatening conditions. Emergency care is provided by a person who is prepared to recognize emergent problems, is able to prioritize, and provide competent skilled care based on professional knowledge or as a prudent layperson. Emergency care is not defined by a practice setting and may be provided within the clinical setting or external to a clinical setting. (Davis et al., 2020, p. 364)

REFERENCE

Davis, W. D., Dowling Evans, D., Fiebig, W., & Lewis, C. L. (2020). Emergency care: Operationalizing the practice through a concept analysis. *Journal of the American Association of Nurse Practitioners*, 32(5), 359–366. https://doi.org/10.1097/JXX.0000000000000229

CHAPTER 3.1

Evolution of the Emergency Nurse Practitioner

Jennifer Wilbeck

INTRODUCTION

Since the inception of the nurse practitioner (NP) role in the mid-1960s, NPs have been providing care for patients experiencing acute illnesses and injuries. Modern definitions of emergency care are built around unscheduled care for acute illnesses, injuries, or exacerbations of chronic conditions (American Academy of Emergency Nurse Practitioners [AAENP], 2018a; American College of Emergency Physicians [ACEP], 2021). When this definition of emergency care is utilized broadly, two constructs emerge:

- NPs have been providing emergency care for decades and even centuries.
- Emergency care does not only occur within the hospital setting.

Rather, the emergency nurse practitioner (ENP) role has evolved in response to healthcare needs similarly to other NP roles (e.g., adult-gerontology and pediatric acute care NP; Peacock et al., 2022). Within the United States, the availability of healthcare providers, access to emergency care, and the need for quality yet cost-effective care amid increasing patient volumes in emergency care settings have informed and shaped the role of the NP in these settings. Prior to the publication of the *Consensus Model for APRN Regulation: Licensure, Accreditation, Certification, and Education* in 2008, NPs with multiple certifications and degrees representing diverse populations provided emergency care in the United States (Hoyt et al., 2018). While the Consensus Model was intended to clarify NP practice, for NPs providing such a unique role in emergency care, the model ultimately presented a challenge for recognition and regulation.

The formal recognition of NPs in emergency care was first supported by the Emergency Nurses Association (ENA) with the 2008 competencies (ENA, 2008). From its inception in 1970, the Emergency Department Nurse Association (which later became the ENA in 1985) supported robust emergency care. It was not until 2004, however, that the ENA developed an APRN task force to specifically support and lead initiatives for ENPs (Hoyt et al., 2018).

The American Nurses Association formally recognized emergency nursing (including both nurses and APRNs) as a specialty in 2011. In the early years of formal emergency NP practice, most NPs were utilized within a fast-track setting within EDs. In this role, NPs were providing care to lower acuity patients such as those presenting with upper respiratory illnesses, mild injuries, or other complaints commonly seen within primary care settings. For NPs working in rural settings and critical access hospitals, however, they were providing stabilizing emergency care to all acuities.

Over time, the NP's role in emergency care grew with the dynamic changes in emergency care delivery. Currently, NPs are utilized in various types of emergency care settings, including diverse geographical locations with a wide range of populations, conditions, and care needs (Pines et al., 2020). These practice settings may include provider roles in triage, fast track, academic/tertiary care, suburban/community EDs, rural emergency settings, urgent care (including telehealth), and solo practice in critical access facilities. Emergency NPs also now provide care in nontraditional, prehospital settings such as emergency medical services (EMS) and mobile integrated services (AAENP, 2022).

ORGANIZATIONAL SUPPORT FOR NURSE PRACTITIONERS IN EMERGENCY CARE

The growth of ENP numbers and diversity of practice was enhanced by efforts from multiple organizations. As the needs of NPs in emergency care were recognized, groups provided the data, answers, and advocacy needed to support both NPs and ongoing patient care. Similarly, as the ENP role expanded, organizations saw continued and evolving opportunities to engage and support the evolving healthcare workforce.

Emergency Nurses Association

The first scope of practice for APRNs in emergency care was initially published by the ENA in 1999 (Cole et al., 1999). With the continued growth of ENP practice, the ENA assembled an NP validation work team to explore and delineate ENP competencies (Hoyt et al., 2010). In collaboration with key emergency physicians and nursing organizations, the ENA hosted stakeholder meetings which ultimately led to the establishment of scientifically derived emergency care competencies for NPs (ENA, 2008). These competencies were updated by the ENA in 2019 (ENA, 2019).

American Nurses Credentialing Center

The first certification for ENPs was offered by the American Nurses Credentialing Center (ANCC) in 2013 as a certification by portfolio. This mechanism for certification was discontinued in November 2017. In total, 124 NPs were certified via this process (Hoyt et al., 2018).

American Academy of Emergency Nurse Practitioners

Initially formed in 2014, the AAENP focused from inception on providing the structure needed to both support and further the ENP role. In response to national needs for standardized ENP education and formal recognition of the ENP role, the AAENP has developed the following:

- ENP scope and standards of practice (AAENP, 2016), endorsed by the ENA
- ENP competencies within the context of practice standards (AAENP, 2018b), offering a framework for assessing the progression of competence from novice to expert
- The definition of emergency care for nurse practitioners (AAENP, 2018a)
- Validation standards for educational programs (AAENP, 2020)
- Publication of the *Emergency Nurse Practitioner Core Curriculum* text (Holleran & Campo, 2022)
- Advocacy for a national certification exam recognizing ENP knowledge

American Academy of Nurse Practitioners Certification Board

Built upon the original ENA competencies for ENP practice, a national practice analysis was initially undertaken by the American Academy of Nurse Practitioners Certification Board in 2016 (Tyler et al., 2018). This analysis guided the development of the ENP certification exam initially offered in January 2017.

GRADUATE ACADEMIC PROGRAMS

Specialized graduate academic programs preparing ENPs did not exist until the 1990s. Prior to dedicated programs, ENPs received on-the-job training via direct mentorship by physicians. In 1994, UT Houston began offering the first ENP program. By April 2018, there were 10 graduate-level programs in the United States specifically preparing NPs for emergency practice (AAENP, 2018c). A total of 16 academic programs existed in May 2023. **Figure 1** provides a summary of milestones in the growth of the ENP role.

With increased NP utilization in emergency care settings, academic programs have expanded to offer dedicated preparation for NPs who intend to practice in emergency care. While there are multiple pathways for an NP to develop specialized emergency care expertise, the most direct educational pathway is through graduate or postgraduate academic ENP programs. The ENP specialty, as currently defined by the *Consensus Model for APRN Regulation* (APRN Consensus Work Group & the National Council of State Boards of Nursing APRN Advisory Committee, 2008), builds upon initial preparation as a family nurse practitioner (FNP). Academic preparation across the life span and acuity continuums prepares NPs for emergency care to patients presenting with diverse and undifferentiated presentations and is supported by physician colleagues (Marco et al., 2021). As the ENP certification is offered as a specialty beyond that of the population, the family population offers the most robust and appropriate basis for education (AAENP, 2018c). While recent years have seen an increasing complexity of

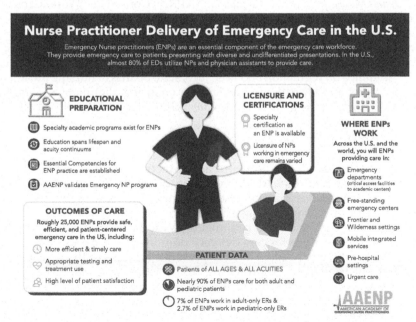

FIGURE 1: Infographic depicting the emergency nurse practitioner role, reproduced with permission from the American Academy of Emergency Nurse Practitioners.

patient conditions, the number of patients requiring acute and resuscitative care pales in comparison to those with primary care and less severe illness and injury (Wu & Darracq, 2021).

CHALLENGES TO EMERGENCY NURSE PRACTITIONER PRACTICE

Despite the expansion of and advocacy for the ENP role, challenges to practice continue to exist. Acknowledgment of the ENP specialty is complicated by the lack of uniformity among regulators, health insurance providers, and employers (Wilbeck et al., 2022). The continued lack of understanding of the NP's role in emergency care challenges the ability to capture potential benefits for patients and healthcare systems (Sanford, 2022). While some challenges have been resolved with intentional collaborations, others persist.

Competencies

As organizations continued to explore the most appropriate utilization of ENPs, having two different sets of competencies for NPs in emergency care (the 2018 AAENP practice standards and 2019 ENA competencies) propagated the confusion surrounding the ENP role. A singular version of ENP competencies was needed to more clearly delineate essential ENP knowledge, skills, and abilities. Working together, the AAENP and ENA ENP Competencies Work Group released a merged set of ENP competencies in 2021 derived from the existing two sets of competencies (Davis et al., 2022). Ultimately, the most recent ENP competencies (AAENP & ENA, 2021) were endorsed by the National Organization of Nurse Practitioner Faculties in March 2022.

Licensure

The *Consensus Model for APRN Regulation* (APRN Consensus Work Group & the National Council of State Boards of Nursing APRN Advisory Committee, 2008) clearly states that state licensing boards of nursing should not regulate practice at the specialty level. However, there is no current framework for nursing regulatory bodies to recognize, acknowledge, or license NP specialty practice (Wilbeck et al., 2022). In the absence of national guidance on regulation and licensure, state boards of nursing are left to independently interpret and identify mechanisms for ensuring alignment and accessibility to specialty NP care. This is perhaps the greatest challenge and threat to the ENP role.

CONTINUED EVOLUTION AND GROWTH

From its origins to today, the numbers and practice patterns have expanded in response to healthcare needs and the evolution of care delivery models. The combined effects of increased utilization of the ED for urgent and primary care, limited access to care, and physician shortages in certain geographical areas have provided increased opportunities for NPs. In conjunction with the evolution and growth of the NP professions, the locations for care delivery demonstrate the widespread response of NPs to broad healthcare needs. The ENP presence remains within diverse settings, including but not limited to EDs (ranging from critical access facilities to tertiary care centers), urgent care, free standing emergency centers, prehospital care/emergency medical response, mobile integrated services, and observation medicine units (AAENP, 2022; Wu & Darracq, 2021). The utilization of NPs in the delivery of emergency care appears greater within rural settings than in urban areas (Hall et al., 2018).

Within emergency care delivery in the United States, NPs provide excellent care. Multiple benefits of care provided by ENPs have been recently demonstrated, including patient satisfaction, resource utilization, reducing ED length of stay and return visits, and improving patient and system outcomes (Mafi et al., 2022; Wilbeck et al., 2023). **Figure 2** provides a graphic summary of the care delivered by NP in emergency care settings across the United States.

Currently, almost 80% of EDs in the United States utilize NPs and physician assistants (PAs) to provide care (Wu & Darracq, 2021). Multiple studies have demonstrated

Mid-1960s	NP role emerges
1994	UT Houston School of Nursing offers first master's ENP program
1999	ENA develops APRN Scope of Practice
2004	ENA develops APRN Task Force
2008	*Consensus Model for APRN Regulation* is published
2011	ANA recognizes emergency nursing (RN and APRN) as a specialty
2013	ANCC launches ENP certification by portfolio
2014	American Academy of Emergency Nurse Practitioners (AAENP) is established
2016	*ENP Scopes and Standards* published by AAENP
	AANPCB conducts national practice analysis of NPs in emergency care
2017	AANPCB launches certification by examination
	ANCC discontinues ENP certification by portfolio
2018	AAENP publishes *ENP Competencies as Practice Standards*
2019	ENA releases updated ENP Competencies
2020	AAENP establishes Program Validation process
2021	AAENP and ENA release unified set of ENP competencies
2022	First edition of the *ENP Core Curriculum* published (Springer Publishing)
2023	AAENP reaffirms support for ENP as a population

FIGURE 2: Timeline of the evolving emergency nurse practitioner role.

AAENP, American Academy of Emergency Nurse Practitioners; AANPCB, American Academy of Nurse Practitioners Certification Board; ANA, American Nurses Association; ANCC, American Nurses Credentialing Center; ENA, Emergency Nurses Association; ENP, emergency nurse practitioner; NP, nurse practitioner.

continued growth and evolution among NPs working in emergency care. The following developments took place in recent years:

- From 2012 to 2018, ENP numbers increased by nearly 9% (Marco et al., 2021).
- Between 2019 and 2022, the number of NPs working in emergency settings increased by over 50%, totaling approximately 27,000 NPs (American Association of Nurse Practitioners [AANP] 2019, 2022).

It is anticipated that the ENP presence will experience an 8% annual growth rate through 2030 (Marco et al., 2021).

SUMMARY

NPs have demonstrated that they are an integral part of the emergency care workforce in the United States. Based on decades of positive outcomes and evolving roles that continue to support safe and efficient emergency care delivery, recent projections are that NPs will increasingly provide emergency care in the coming years. With increasing national ED workforce needs, ENPs are now participating to a greater extent within emergency medicine teams in the delivery of collaborative emergency care. The growth of targeted emergency NP educational programs, organizational advocacy efforts, and the healthcare landscape have positioned ENPs to continue answering workforce and patient care needs in the provision of quality and safe care for diverse patients and presentations. Support of academic ENP preparation and certification from physician colleagues (Marco et al., 2021) offers additional opportunities to continue high-quality care delivery.

With increasing numbers and presence of NPs in emergency care, continued research assessing patient outcomes and health system benefits are needed to further the ENP role in satisfying population needs. To support future uniformity in education and licensure and in efforts to further clarify the role and recognition of the ENP, exploration of transitioning the ENP to the NP population rather than a specialty is progressing (Wilbeck et al., 2022). In 2023, AAENP noted ". . . that the patient population served by the ENP represents a unique and significantly differentiated set of competencies and behaviors from other APRN population foci. Therefore, in collaboration with our national colleagues and regulatory stakeholders, AAENP supports the development of an ENP population" (AAENP, 2023). While the next placement of the ENP role on the APRN Consensus Model remains to be seen, the delivery of safe and quality emergency care by NPs will unquestionably continue in the coming years.

REFERENCES

American Academy of Emergency Nurse Practitioners. (2016). *Scope and standards for emergency nurse practitioner practice.* https://aaenp.memberclicks.net/assets/docs/aaenp_scope_and_standards.pdf

American Academy of Emergency Nurse Practitioners. (2018a, April). *Emergency care definition.* https://www.aaenp-natl.org/assets/docs/emergency_care_definition_8.7.18.pdf

American Academy of Emergency Nurse Practitioners. (2018b). *Practice standards for the emergency nurse practitioner specialty.* https://www.aaenp-natl.org/assets/docs/practice_standards_for_the_emergency_nurse_practitioner.pdf

American Academy of Emergency Nurse Practitioners. (2018c, April). Emergency Nurse Practitioner Practice Data: Executive Summary. https://www.aaenp-natl.org/assets/docs/enppractice_data_exec_summary_final.pdf

American Academy of Emergency Nurse Practitioners. (2020). *Standards for academic program validation.* https://www.aaenp-natl.org/assets/Standards%20for%20ENP%20Academic%20Program%20Validation%20%285%29.pdf

American Academy of Emergency Nurse Practitioners. (2022). *Role of nurse practitioners in emergency medical services: An AAENP position statement.* https://aaenp.memberclicks.net/assets/docs/NP%20in%20EMS%20Role%20Position%20Statement_Approved051022.pdf

American Academy of Emergency Nurse Practitioners. (2023). *Re-envisioning the emergency nurse practitioner role.* https://aaenp.memberclicks.net/assets/docs/ENP%20Role%20Position%20Statement%20revison%20proposed%20to%20BOD%202023%20v2.pdf

American Academy of Emergency Nurse Practitioners & Emergency Nurses Association. (2021). *Emergency nurse practitioner competencies.* https://aaenp.memberclicks.net/assets/docs/ENPcompetencies_FINAL2.pdf

American Association of Nurse Practitioners. (2019). *AANP nurse practitioner compensation report.* https://storage.aanp.org/www/documents/no-index/research/2019-NPSample-Survey-Report.pdf 4

American Association of Nurse Practitioners. (2022). *NP fact sheet.* https://storage.aanp.org/www/documents/NPFacts__111022.pdf

American College of Emergency Physicians. (2021). *Definition of emergency medicine.* acep.org/pateient-care/policy-statements/definition-of-emergency-medicine

APRN Consensus Work Group & the National Council of State Boards of Nursing APRN Advisory Committee. (2008). *Consensus model for APRN regulation: Licensure, accreditation, certification & education.* https://www.nursingworld.org/~4aa7d9/globalassets/certification/aprn_consensus_model_report_7-7-08.pdf

Cole, F., Ramirez, E., & Luna-Gonzales, H. (1999). *Scope of practice for the nurse practitioner in the emergency care setting.* Emergency Nurses Association.

Davis, W. D., Hallman, M. G., Denke, N. J., House, D. T., Switzer, D. F., & Wilbeck, J. (2022). A collaboration to unify emergency nurse practitioner competencies. *Journal for Nurse Practitioners, 18*(8), 889–892. https://doi-org.libproxy.usouthal.edu/10.1016/j.nurpra.2022.06.014

Emergency Nurses Association. (2008). *Competencies for nurse practitioners in emergency care.*

Emergency Nurses Association. (2019). *Emergency nurse practitioner competencies.* https://www.ena.org/docs/default-source/resource-library/practice-resources/other/practitioner-competencies.pdf?sfvrsn=db39b977_10

Hall, M. K., Burns, K., Carius, M., Erickson, M., Hall, J., & Venkatesh, A. (2018). State of the national emergency department workforce: Who provides care where? *Annals of Emergency Medicine, 72*(3), 302–307.

Holleran, R., & Campo, T. (2022). *Emergency nurse practitioner core curriculum.* Springer Publishing.

Hoyt, K. S., Coyne, E. A., Ramirez, E. G., Peard, A. S., Gisness, C., & Gacki-Smith, J. (2010). Nurse practitioner Delphi study: Competencies for practice in emergency care. *Journal of Emergency Nursing, 36*(5), 439–449. https://doi-org.libproxy.usouthal.edu/10.1016/j.jen.2010.05.001

Hoyt, K. S., Evans, D., Wilbeck, J., Ramirez, E., Agan, D., Tyler, D., & Schumann, L. (2018). Appraisal of the emergency nurse practitioner specialty role. *Journal of the American Association of Nurse Practitioners, 30*, 551–559.

Mafi, J. N., Chen, A., Guo, R., Choi, K., Smulowitz, P., Tseng, C-H., Ladapo, J. A., & Landon, B. E. (2022). US emergency care patterns among nurse practitioners and physician assistants compared with physicians: A cross-sectional analysis. *BMJ Open, 12*(4), e055138. https://doi.org/10.1136/bmjopen-2021-055138

Marco, C. A., Courtney, D. M., Ling, L. J., Salsberg, E., Reisdorff, E. J., Gallahue, F. E., Suter, R. E., Muelleman, R., Chappell, B., Evans, D. D., Vafaie, N., & Richwine, C. (2021). The emergency medicine physician workforce: Projections for 2030. *Annals of Emergency Medicine, 78*(6), 726–737. https://doi.org/10.1016/j.annemergmed.2021.05.029

Peacock, A., Blakely, K., Maes, C., Henson, A., DiGiulio, M., & Henderson, M. J. (2022). Adult-gerontology nurse practitioners: A discussion of scope and expertise. *The Journal for Nurse Practitioners, 18*, 1037–1045.

Pines, J. M., Zocchi, M. S., Ritsema, T. S., Polansky, M., Bedolla, J., Venkat, A., & for the US Acute Care Solutions Research Group. (2020). The impact of advanced practice provider staffing on emergency department care: Productivity, flow, safety, and experience. *Academic Emergency Medicine, 27*(11), 1089–1099.

Sanford, K. (2022, June). Challenges to the essential roles of advanced practice providers. *NEJM Catalyst: Innovations in Care Delivery, 3*(6). https://doi.org/10.1056/CAT.22.0146

Tyler, D. O., Hoyt, K. S., Evans, D. D., Schumann, L., Ramirez, E., Wilbeck, J., & Agan, D. (2018). Emergency nurse practitioner practice analysis: Report and implications of the findings. *Journal of the American Association of Nurse Practitioners, 30*(10), 560–569. https://doi.org/10.1097/JXX.0000000000000118

Wilbeck, J., Davis, W., Tyler, D., Schumann, L., & Kapu, A. (2023). Analysis of nurse practitioner practice in U.S. emergency departments: Evidence supporting the educational preparation, credentialing, scope of practice & outcomes. *Journal of the American Association of Nurse Practitioners, 35*(6), 373–379. Online ahead of print, May 5.

Wilbeck, J., Schumann, L., Comer, A., & Davis, W. (2022). Consideration of the emergency nurse practitioner as a population within the advanced practice registered nurse consensus model: A SWOT analysis. *Journal of the American Association of Nurse Practitioners, 34*(10), 1126.

Wu, F., & Darracq, M. A. (2021). Comparing physician assistant and nurse practitioner practice in U.S. emergency departments, 2010–2017. *Western Journal of Emergency Medicine, 22*(5), 1150–1155.

CHAPTER 4.1

Full Practice Authority

April Kapu
Valerie Fuller

INTRODUCTION

The development of the first nurse practitioner (NP) program in 1965 by Drs. Loretta Ford and Henry Silver ushered in a new and transformative role for advanced practice nursing. Initially conceived as a pediatric primary care role, it has expanded to include multiple other populations and specialties, including the emergency nurse practitioner (ENP; Fuller & McCauley, 2023). Since its earliest beginnings, NPs have sought to provide patient-centered care that utilizes the full scope of their education, certification, licensure, and training—a concept known as full practice authority (FPA).

As defined by the American Nurses Association (2020), FPA is "an APRN's ability to utilize knowledge, skills, and judgment to practice to the full extent of his or her education and training." The American Association of Nurse Practitioners (AANP) has further defined FPA as "the authorization of NPs to evaluate patients, diagnose, order and interpret diagnostic tests, and initiate and manage treatments—including prescribing medications—under the exclusive licensure authority of the state board of nursing" (AANP, 2022). Currently, 27 states, the District of Columbia, and two U.S. territories (Guam and the Northern Mariana Islands) have FPA for NPs. **Figure 1** shows which states are known as FPA states and which have reduced or restricted practice, collectively referred to as "non-FPA" states.

In 2008, the APRN Consensus Work Group, in collaboration with the National Council of State Boards of Nursing (NCSBN) APRN Advisory Committee, introduced the *Consensus Model for APRN Regulation: Licensure, Accreditation, Certification, and Education*. The goal of the Consensus Model was to address the lack of definitions related to APRN roles, lack of standardization in APRN preparation programs, proliferation of APRN specialties, and the lack of common legal recognition across jurisdictions (APRN Consensus Work Group, 2008). The Consensus Model includes the four recognized APRN roles (certified NP, certified nurse midwife, clinical nurse specialist, and certified registered nurse anesthetist) and six population foci (family, adult-gerontology [acute and primary], women's health/gender related, neonatal, pediatrics [acute and primary], and psychiatric/mental health; see **Figure 2**). The major elements for each role include state recognition of each of

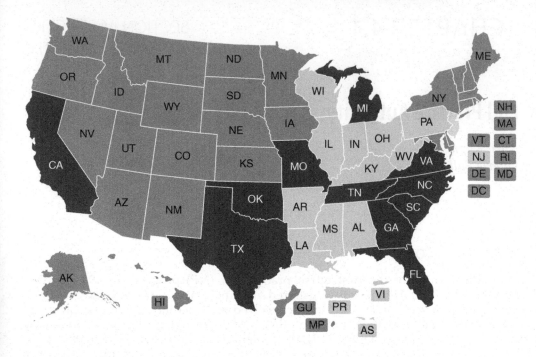

Full Practice: State practice and licensure laws permit all NPs to evaluate patients; diagnose, order and interpret diagnostic tests; and initiate and manage treatments, including prescribing medications and controlled substances, under the exclusive licensure authority of the state board of nursing. This is the model recommended by the National Academy of Medicine, formerly called the Institute of Medicine, and the National Council of State Boards of Nursing.

Reduced Practice: State practice and licensure laws reduce the ability of NPs to engage in at least one element of NP practice. State law requires a career-long regulated collaborative agreement with another health provider in order for the NP to provide patient care, or it limits the setting of one or more elements of NP practice.

Restricted Practice: State practice and licensure laws restrict the ability of NPs to engage in at least one element of NP practice. State law requires career-long supervision, delegation or team management by another health provider in order for the NP to provide patient care.

FIGURE 1: 2023 Nurse practitioner state practice environment.

Source: American Association of Nurse Practitioners. (2023). *2023 Nurse practitioner state practice environment.* https://storage.aanp.org/www/documents/advocacy/State-Practice-Environment.pdf

the four roles, APRN title for each role, licensure as an RN and APRN, graduate or postgraduate education from an accredited program, certification at an advanced level that is maintained, independent practice, and independent prescribing (APRN Consensus Work Group, NCSBN APRN Advisory Committee, 2008).

As outlined in the Consensus Model, licensure by boards of nursing (BONs) is regulated at the level of the APRN role and population foci. APRN specialties, which focus on practice beyond the role and population focus, are not regulated by BONs.

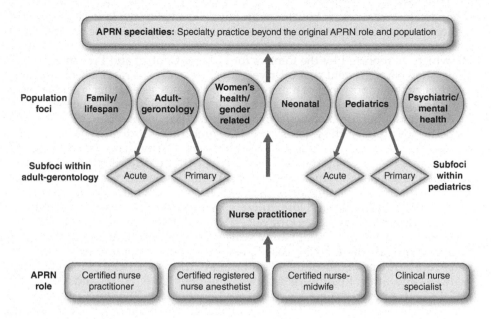

FIGURE 2: APRN regulatory model.

Source: Adapted from NCSBN. (2008). *Consensus model for APRN regulation: Licensure, accreditation, certification and education.* https://www.ncsbn.org/public-files/Consensus_Model_for_APRN_Regulation_July_2008.pdf

THE CASE FOR FULL PRACTICE AUTHORITY

Despite national standards for accredited education, training, and board certification, the licensure authority to practice lies with the state. Each state's rules and regulations for licensure and renewal can vary, creating significant variations in practice from state to state. "FPA is the authorization of NPs to evaluate patients, diagnose, order and interpret diagnostic tests and initiate and manage treatments—including prescribing medications—under the exclusive licensure authority of the state board of nursing" (AANP, 2023b). In states with FPA, there is an increase in consistency in practice as practice aligns with education and training. Studies have correlated FPA with better health outcomes, an increase in the workforce, and increased access to care (Yang et al., 2021). For example, Arizona adopted FPA in 2001. From 2002 to 2007, the number of NPs increased by 53% across all counties, with the biggest increase in counties classified as rural–rural, in which there was a 73% increase (Eng et al., 2011). And year over year, Arizona has increased in rankings for overall health outcomes to 21 out of 50 in 2021 (America's Health Rankings, 2021). In 2021, the healthiest states were New Hampshire, Massachusetts, Vermont, Connecticut, and Hawaii, all FPA states. The states with the lowest rankings were Louisiana, Mississippi, Arkansas, West Virginia, and Alabama, all restricted, non-FPA, states (America's Health Rankings, 2021). Data related to workforce and outcomes are important to track once a state adopts FPA. The correlation demonstrates that FPA can be a significant precursor to addressing the nation's healthcare access and workforce challenges.

Access, health outcomes, and workforce are among the nation's greatest challenges in healthcare. In 2023, the Department of Health and Human Services (2023) reported 99 million Americans lack access to primary care, while 160 million Americans lack access to mental health services. A Mercer (2021) analysis indicated a shortage of up to

3.2 million healthcare workers by 2026, with physicians being the largest group. Even more concerning is that chronic comorbidities, such as obesity, heart disease, and diabetes, continue to escalate (Stierman et al., 2021). All these issues have a profound impact on EDs, which, as reported by the Centers for Disease Control and Prevention (CDC, 2021), have shown a consistent year-over-year increase in census rates. These issues not only emphasize the importance of managing chronic diseases effectively and preventing them through community-based health services but also highlight the need for an adequate number of qualified and effective healthcare providers within EDs.

Organizations and health systems are hiring qualified NPs to provide high-quality care for patients in the community and in the EDs. The evidence is clear that NPs can provide care that is comparable to physicians with no difference in patient care outcomes. A Liu et al. (2020) study of 806,434 patients who were reassigned to NPs in the Veterans Affairs (VA) health system, across 530 VAs, demonstrated similar patient care outcomes to physicians and less utilization of comparable costs. In addition, as consumers of care, patients are seeking out NPs as evidenced by over one billion visits to NPs each year (AANP, 2023b). Innovative efforts to meet patients "where they are" are expanding through an increased presence of NPs in community-based clinics, home care services, telehealth, school-based clinics, tribal clinics, skilled nursing facilities, and other healthcare settings. Buerhaus et al. (2018) and DesRoches et al. (2017) both found that among Medicare beneficiaries, there was a lower risk of preventable hospitalization with primary care NPs practicing in the community, and there was a direct correlation to the reduction of the use of ED services.

Many acute and primary care NPs work in EDs with continued education training, and many seek additional advanced certification in emergency care. There are NPs working in critical access and rural EDs often as solo providers. ED NPs (ENPs) not only provide stabilization and acute resuscitation but also facilitate coordination of care across large networks, including transfers to larger hospital systems and specialists.

Given the issues facing access to care and the known data supporting the increase in access to care, expansion of the workforce, and impact on patient care outcomes, there is a compelling case for states to move to update licensure laws to allow NPs to work to the extent of their education and training. Yang et al. (2021) emphasize the impact that unnecessary, outdated state licensure laws can have on the workforce, the distribution of the workforce across the state, utilization of healthcare services, costs, and quality of care. The case for removing barriers to NP practice has been outlined on numerous occasions, as noted in Robert Wood Johnson's *Charting Nursing's Future* report and in *The Future of Nursing 2020–2030* report (National Academy of Medicine [NAM], 2021; Robert Wood Johnson Foundation [RWJF], 2017). Simply put, evidence has demonstrated that FPA will offer residents within each state the full benefits of NP care and enable NPs to improve healthcare access, quality, and value (NAM, 2021).

RESTRICTED PRACTICE AUTHORITY

There are several different categories of state licensure restrictions that preclude an NP from FPA. The most common restrictive limitation among the 23 non-FPA states is a mandatory, career-long contract with one or more physicians. The terms of these contracts vary from state to state without clear rationale. For example, in Tennessee, the contracted physician must make a site visit in person monthly and perform a retrospective review of 20% of the NP's patient records or charts, commonly known as "chart review." For other states, chart review may not be required, or the percentage varies as low as 5%. The efficacy of retrospective chart review for the entirety of an NP's career has not been well studied, and its direct impact on patient care is limited in that the chart review occurs well after the patient visit. In some states, physicians may charge a fee for chart review and other contractual obligations, and these fees can be unregulated, creating a financial barrier for NPs and health systems.

Beyond state-mandated contracts, there are other types of restrictions such as prescribing limitations, usually related to controlled substances or specific categories of controlled substances. There can be geographical, setting, or population-specific restrictions. Examples include states where NPs can have FPA in rural communities but not in urban areas or where an NP can have FPA in primary care settings but not in acute care settings. Of the 23 reduced or restricted practice authority states, 21 require a mandated contract with a physician, 12 have prescribing limitations, three have geographical or population-specific limitations, and four have APRN oversight by a professional board outside of nursing (AANP, 2023c). All restrictions create additional, unnecessary administrative work, such as record keeping, contract management, accounts payable, staffing, and technical infrastructure. For NPs working in the ED, where care discussions are often at the time of service, the retrospective review processes can be unnecessarily duplicative and costly not only for the ENP but, oftentimes, also for the healthcare system. Lastly, in four non-FPA states having an additional professional board, other than nursing, oversight and regulation of NP practice can be problematic.

Institutional Restrictions

It is important to note that FPA is regulated at the state level based on state licensure. A clinic, hospital, or other healthcare organization may have additional limitations related to an NP's scope of practice. For example, a hospital's medical staff bylaws may have additional rules or restrictions that impact the NP's practice within the organization. For institutions that require credentialing and privileging approval to provide patient care, the medical staff rules and regulations must be abided by for the NP to practice within the facility.

Most EDs are associated with a hospital or health system that requires credentialing and privileging. A 2021 study examining the utilization of NPs in states with FPA suggests that restrictions on privileges at the system level were most frequently seen with NPs who practice in critical care, urgent care, EDs, and specialty area practices as compared to primary care settings and concluded that FPA has not necessarily led to fewer restrictions at the organizational level (Zwilling et al., 2021). This underscores the importance of understanding both state FPA and organizational policies to navigate the scope of practice effectively.

COVID-19 PANDEMIC

During the COVID-19 pandemic, 20 non-FPA states' governors issued executive orders waiving restrictions such as management of contracts, chart review, on-site visits, and/or setting and population limitations. Largely, this measure was to increase access to care and optimize the healthcare workforce. The AANP maintained a webpage outlining the terms of each state's executive order, including the dates of implementation and expiration (AANP, 2023a). It is uncertain as to the reason for returning to previous restrictions upon expiration of executive orders. Yuanhong et al. (2020) stated that practice authority should be based on outcomes, such as access, quality, and cost of care, and that the return to practice restrictions must align with empirical evidence (2020). Interestingly, during the pandemic years 2020 to 2023, five states—Massachusetts, Delaware, Kansas, New York, and Utah—moved to FPA.

ENPs, like many other healthcare providers, demonstrate a remarkable commitment to ensuring access to healthcare for their communities. They played an instrumental role in expanding ED services, launching hospital-to-home programs,

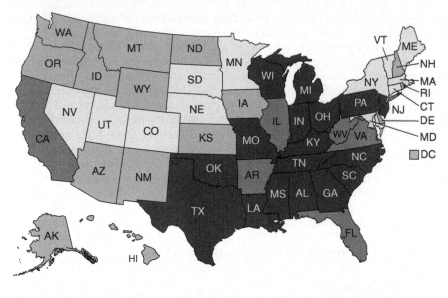

■ **Full practice* without transition to practice**

□ **Full practice* with transition to practice**

■ **Reduced practice* or restricted practice* with transition to practice**

■ **Reduced practice* or restricted practice* without transition to practice**

[Washington, D.C. is included in this visual summary only.]

AR: 6,240 hours postlicensure practice period

CA: 3-year or 4,600-hour postlicensure practice period

CO: 750-hour postlicensure practice period

CT: 3-year and a minimum of 2,000-hour postlicensure practice period

FL: 3,000-hour postlicensure practice period (primary care practice as defined)

IL: 4,000-hour postlicensure practice period and 250 hours of CE/training units; physician consultation required when prescribing schedule II controlled substances and benzodiazepines

MA: 2-year postlicensure practice period for independent prescribing authority

MD: 18-month postlicensure practice period

ME: 24-month postlicensure practice period

MN: 2,080-hour postlicensure practice period

NE: 2,000-hour postlicensure practice period

NV: 2-year or 2,000-hour postlicensure practice period

NY: 3,600-hour postlicensure practice period

SD: 1,040-hour postlicensure practice period

UT: 1,000-hour mentorship for NPs in independent solo practice who have less than one year or 2,000 hours of experience as an APRN for prescribing Schedule II controlled substances

VA: 5-year full-time postlicensure practice period

VT: 2-year and 2,400-hour post-licensure practice period

WV: 3-year postlicensure practice period; excludes Schedule I controlled substances

*As defined by the American Association of Nurse Practitioners. https://www.aanp.org/advocacy/state/state-practice-environment

FIGURE 3: Full practice authority and non-full practice authority states with transition to practice requirements.

Source: Haney, B. (2023). 35th annual APRN legislative update. *The Nurse Practitioner, 48*(1), 20–47. https://doi.org/10.1097/01. NPR.0000903012.03553.a4

initiating hotlines for COVID-19-related calls, and establishing off-site testing centers to decrease the ED testing volume. These efforts were crucial in ensuring patients received timely and effective care while minimizing the spread of the virus. The FPA restriction waivers were essential to supporting these innovative effects streamlining care amid the substantial access and care challenges throughout the pandemic. Poghosyan et al. (2022, p. 33) emphasize "state policymakers should utilize the momentum created by the pandemic to permanently eliminate practice barriers."

TRANSITION TO PRACTICE

Transition to practice (TTP) periods are state-mandated regulations that require an NP to work under the supervision of another healthcare provider (physician or, in some states, an APRN) for a defined number of hours or years before being granted FPA. In states with FPA and a TTP mandate, NPs will obtain FPA after the TTP requirement has been satisfied. TTPs are not uniformly required nor defined across states, and there is no evidence to suggest that these restrictions improve patient care or provide public protection. These regulations have created unintended consequences for patients and providers alike. For example, in Connecticut, APRNs can move to FPA after the completion of a TTP under the supervision of a physician licensed in Connecticut after 3 years with at least 2,000 hours (Connecticut, 2020). However, an APRN with FPA is not allowed to provide the state-mandated supervision of a newly licensed Connecticut APRN during the 3-year period. Additionally, for APRNs moving to Connecticut from out of state, even though they may have over 3 years of experience, they must start at zero and obtain 3 years of TTP, including 2,000 practice hours within Connecticut under the supervision of a state-licensed physician.

TTPs restrict patient access to care, particularly in rural areas, and NPs may experience significant challenges in finding and retaining supervising providers. In addition, NPs are less apt to move into states with more restrictive practice environments, further limiting access to care. For these reasons, Colorado has steadily decreased its TTP; the most recent decrease was in 2020 to 750 supervised hours by a physician or APRN (Colorado, 2020). TTP requirements are seen both in states with FPA and in reduced practice states. **Figure 3** shows these requirements in detail. Unfortunately, removing TTP limitations is challenging. In 2021, Maine attempted to modernize its rules and regulations and remove the TTP period that had been in place for over 20 years. Despite support from the BON, which advocated for its removal, citing decades of safe practice, the legislation was not successful.

SUMMARY

Decades of empirical evidence and scientific research have demonstrated NPs provide high-quality, cost-effective, and efficient healthcare. Overly restrictive state regulations that impede NPs from practicing to the full extent of their education and training result in reduced access to care, limited expansion of the NP workforce, and adverse healthcare outcomes. It is, therefore, crucial that these barriers be eliminated to maximize the benefits of NP practice and ensure access to care.

REFERENCES

American Association of Nurse Practitioners. (2022). *Nurse practitioners*. https://storage.aanp.org/www/documents/research/2022-Data-Integrity-Infographic.pdf
American Association of Nurse Practitioners. (2023a). *COVID-19 state emergency response: Temporarily suspended and waived practice agreement requirements*. https://www.aanp.org/advocacy/state/covid-19-state-emergency-response-temporarily-suspended-and-waived-practice-agreement-requirements

American Association of Nurse Practitioners. (2023b, March). *Issues at a glance: Full practice authority.* https://www.aanp.org/advocacy/advocacy-resource/policy-briefs/issues-full-practice-brief

American Association of Nurse Practitioners. (2023c). *State practice environment.* https://www.aanp.org/advocacy/state

American Nurses Association. (2020, February). *Ana's principles for advanced practice registered nurse (APRN) full practice authority.* https://www.nursingworld.org/~495dca/globalassets/docs/ana/ethics/principles-aprnfullpracticeauthority.pdf

America's Health Rankings. (2021). *2021 annual report.* https://www.americashealthrankings.org/learn/reports/2021-annual-report

APRN Consensus Work Group, National Council of State Boards of Nursing APRN Advisory Committee. (2008). *Consensus model for APRN regulation: Licensure, accreditation, certification & education.* NCSBN. https://ncsbn.org/Consensus_Model_for_APRN_Regulation_July_2008.pdf

Buerhaus, P., Perloff, J., Clarke, S., O'Reilly-Jacob, M., Zolotusky, G., & DesRoches, C. M. (2018). Quality of primary care provided to medicare beneficiaries by nurse practitioners and physicians. *Medical Care, 56*(6), 484–490. https://doi-org./10.1097/MLR.0000000000000908

Centers for Disease Control and Prevention. (2021). *Health, United States, 2020-2021.* https://www.cdc.gov/nchs/data/hus/2020-2021/EdAd.pdf

Connecticut State. (2020). *Department of Health: Practice without a collaborative agreement.* https://portal.ct.gov/DPH/Practitioner-Licensing--Investigations/APRN/APRN-Practice

Department of Health and Human Services. (2023). *Health workforce shortage areas.* https://data.hrsa.gov/topics/health-workforce/shortage-areas

DesRoches, C. M., Clarke, S., Perloff, J., O'Reilly-Jacob, M., & Buerhaus, P. (2017). The quality of primary care provided by nurse practitioners to vulnerable Medicare beneficiaries. *Nursing Outlook, 65*(6), 679–688.

Eng, H. J., Tabor, J., & Hughes, A. (2011). *Arizona rural health workforce trend analysis.* Arizona Area Health Education Centers Program.

Fuller, V. J., & McCauley, P. S. (2023). Role of the acute care nurse practitioner. In *Textbook for the adult-gerontology acute care nurse practitioner: Evidence-based standards of Practice* (pp. 3–10). Springer Publishing Company.

Liu, C. F., Hebert, P. L., Douglas, J. H., Neely, E. L., Sulc, C. A., Reddy, A., & Wong, E. S. (2020). Outcomes of primary care delivery by nurse practitioners: Utilization, cost, and quality of care. *Health Services Research, 55*(2), 178–189.

Mercer. (2021). *US healthcare labor market.* https://www.mercer.us/content/dam/mercer/assets/content-images/north-america/united-states/us-healthcare-news/us-2021-healthcare-labor-market-whitepaper.pdf

National Academy of Medicine. (2021). *The future of nursing 2020-2030: Charting a path to achieve health equity.* https://nam.edu/publications/the-future-of-nursing-2020-2030/

National Council of State Boards of Nursing. (2008). *The Consensus Model for APRN Regulation.* https://www.ncsbn.org/nursing-regulation/practice/aprn/aprn-consensus.page

Poghosyan, L., Pulcini, J., Chan, G., Dunphy, L., Martsoff, G., Greco, K., Todd, B., Brown, S., Fitzgerald, M., McMenamin, A., & Solari-Twadell, A. (2022). State responses to COVID-19: Potential benefits of continuing full practice authority for primary nurse practitioner. *Nursing Outlook, 70*(1), 28–35.

Robert Wood Johnson Foundation. (2017). *Charting nursing's future: Reports that can inform policy and practice.* file:///C:/Users/april/Downloads/rwjf435543.pdf

State of Colorado. (2020). *Colorado General Assembly 74th Session: Sunset nurse practice act.* https://leg.colorado.gov/bills/hb20-1216

Stierman, B., Afful, J., Carroll, M. D., Chen, T., Davy, O., Fink, S., Fryar, C. D., Gu, Q., Hales, C., Hughes, J. P., Ostchega, Y., Storandt, R. J., & Akinbami, L. J. (2021). *National Health and Nutrition Examination Survey 2017–March 2020 prepandemic data files development of files and prevalence estimates for selected health outcomes.* https://stacks.cdc.gov/view/cdc/106273

Yang, B. K., Johantgen, M. E., Trinkoff, A. M., Idzik, S. R., Wince, J., & Tomlinson, C. (2021). State nurse practitioner practice regulations and U.S. health care delivery outcomes: A systematic review. *Medical care research and review: MCRR, 78*(3), 183–196. https://doi-org/10.1177/1077558719901216

Yuanhong, A., Skillman, S. M., & Frogner, B. K. (2020). Is it fair? How to approach professional scope-of-practice policy after the COVID-19 pandemic. *Health Affairs Blog.* https://www.healthaffairs.org/do/10.1377/hblog20200624.983306/full

Zwilling, J., Fiandt, K., & Ahmed, R. (2021). Comparison of rural and urban utilization of nurse practitioners in states with full practice authority. *The Journal for Nurse Practitioners, 17,* 386–393.

CHAPTER 4.2

Emergency Nurse Practitioners as Full Members of the Medical Staff

Melanie Gibbons Hallman
Amanda Comer

INTRODUCTION

Credentialing practices for nurse practitioners (NPs) have evolved and become more refined and specific since the inception of the role in the 1960s. In 2012, to enhance staffing and improve the quality of patient care in hospitals, the Centers for Medicare & Medicaid Services (CMS) revised its regulations to allow NPs to be appointed to a hospital's medical staff. The appointment and privileging of nonphysician practitioners remains a decision of the governing body within each hospital or hospital system. As part of this regulation, the hospital must assure that the medical staff screens and assures credentials of eligible candidates abiding within the professional scope of practice according to state laws and in compliance with medical staff bylaws and governance (Turner, 2012). A need remains to revise bylaws in many hospital organizations to reflect the professional practice of advanced practice providers (APPs) and to expand and elevate their utility within emergency care. Education of individuals implementing credentialing and awarding privileges, determining hospital board appointments, and enhancing understanding of the NP role by physician medical staff could improve the appointment of NPs as full members of the medical staff. In turn, this could lead to NP positions on hospital boards, medical staff membership and committees, and other hospital committees (Pittman et al., 2020).

MEDICAL STAFF CREDENTIALING

Medical staff credentialing is required for anyone providing treatment, care, or services at a medical level of care and decision-making (The Joint Commission, 2017). The purpose of the credentialing process is to assure that providers have completed training, hold active licensure, and have the qualifications and ability to provide medical care within their specialty. Credentialing holds healthcare workers to an equal standard. Organizational or hospital bylaws should specify a credentialing process and requirements for granting approval by a governing body. This process should also delineate steps for limiting the practice of healthcare workers not in compliance with credentialing guidelines or displaying unsatisfactory standards of care (Patel & Sharma, 2022). Approval of privileges must be granted by medical staff governance prior to initiating direct care. Individual healthcare organizations are required to decide whether an NP is "An individual who is licensed and qualified to direct or provide care, treatment, and services in accordance with state law and regulation, applicable federal law and regulation, and organizational policy" (The Joint Commission, 2017). Some organizations only allow the Doctor of Medicine (MD) and Doctor of Osteopathy (DO) to be members of the organized medical staff. Other hospitals or clinics allow NPs and other licensed independent practitioners to be a part of the organized medical staff.

EMERGENCY NURSE PRACTITIONERS AND MEDICAL STAFF CREDENTIALING

Emergency nurse practitioners (ENPs) have much to offer when appointed as full members of the medical staff. The American Academy of Emergency Nurse Practitioners (AAENP) developed and implemented a meticulous standardized process for validation of population-based NP academic programs (Davis et al., 2023). This established validation process structures ENP academic education, assuring sound academic processes for didactic and clinical educational instruction. The 2021 ENP competencies reflect established evidence-based ENP practice that orchestrates the delivery of safe, quality patient care. These competencies support regulatory frameworks, credentialing, and reimbursements (Davis et al., 2022). ENP competencies and the successful completion of an AAENP-validated academic program provide a compass for advanced practice nurses seeking employment in emergency care and a road map of expectations for organizations employing ENP-prepared advanced practice nurses when determining medical staff appointment and delineation of privileges. ENPs are best prepared to navigate and interpret the complex matrix of specific education, competencies, certification, and practice essentials that underpin and scaffold the ENP's role in emergency care. ENPs, as full members of the medical staff, are capable to discern qualifications and make knowledgeable recommendations for the appointment of ENP members to the medical staff, just as physicians are prepared to discern the qualification of their professional colleagues according to specialty, preparation, and practice. Since ENPs are also licensed RNs, prior experiences in nursing roles and healthcare implementation allow them a unique and informed level of global healthcare understanding uncommon to most other healthcare professions.

REFERENCES

Davis, W. D., Denke, N., Hallman, M. G., House, D., Switzer, D. F., & Wilbeck, J. (2022). Collaboration yields 2021 ENP competencies. *Advanced Emergency Nursing Journal, 44*(2), 75–77. https://doi.org/10.1097/TM E.0000000000000411

Davis, W. D., Hallman, M. G., & Wilbeck, J. (2023). Aligning emergency nurse practitioner programs using a national validation process. *The Journal for Nurse Practitioners, 19*(7). https://doi.org/10.1016/j.nurpr a.2023.104653

Patel, R., & Sharma, S. (2022, October). Credentialing. *StatPearls* [Internet]. StatPearls Publishing. [Updated 2022 Oct 24]. https://www.ncbi.nlm.nih.gov/books/NBK519504/

Pittman, P., Leach, B., Everett, C., Han, X., & McElroy, D. (2020). NP and PA privileging in acute care settings: Do scope of practice laws matter? *Medical Care Research and Review, 77*(2), 112–120. https://doi.or g/10.1177/1077558718760333

The Joint Commission. (2017, May 12). *Medical staff standards.* Hospital and Hospital Clinics. https://ww w.jointcommission.org/standards/standard-faqs/hospital-and-hospital-clinics/medical-staff-ms/000 002124/

Turner, S. A. (2012). CMS broadens concept of hospital "medical staff" to provide greater opportunities for nurses and other nonphysician practitioners. *Geriatric Nursing, 33*(4), 302–303. https://doi.org/10.1 016/j.gerinurse.2012.06.003

CHAPTER 4.3

Emergency Nurse Practitioners and Emergency Medical Services

Bradley Goettl
Chivas Guillote

INTRODUCTION

Evolution of Nurse Practitioners in the Modern Emergency Medical Services System

In the past decade, more and more healthcare is being provided outside the walls of healthcare facilities. Nurse practitioners (NPs) have increasingly become integrated into emergency medical services (EMS) systems around the world. As early as 2008, approximately 6% of U.S. NPs involved in emergency care reported working in the prehospital environment. Several factors have influenced this transition, including the increasing recognition of NPs' ability to provide emergency care and the increased demand for accessible healthcare. The range of opportunities available for NPs within the EMS landscape continues to expand. This chapter will explore the evolving role of NPs in EMS and in the out-of-hospital environment.

BACKGROUND

The National Association of EMS Physicians (NAEMSP) is a professional organization dedicated to advancing EMS through education, research, and advocacy (NAEMSP, 2023). The NAEMSP formed an interprofessional advanced practice providers task force. As a result, they issued a position statement recognizing the value of EMS NPs and their ability to augment and support the role of the medical director (Wright et al., 2021). The statement highlighted that EMS NPs providing prehospital clinical care should undergo additional training beyond standard NP education to achieve competence in prehospital care. The roles and functions that NPs can perform include assisting with protocol development, quality assurance, and improvement; education and training; research; direct patient care for patients with varying acuity levels; consulting for EMS crews; participating in community paramedicine programs; assisting with various leadership functions; and acting as liaisons between the EMS system and hospitals.

The American Academy of Emergency Nurse Practitioners (AAENP, 2022) issued a statement affirming that "Nurse Practitioners are uniquely positioned to provide and direct care of the patient within a multidisciplinary EMS system." In this statement, the AAENP acknowledged that NPs are increasingly becoming integral members of the EMS system, assuming vital responsibilities such as responding to 911 calls, facilitating interfacility transport, participating in mobile integrated health programs, and driving population health initiatives. Within the EMS system, NPs possess the authority to directly administer comprehensive care, including advanced interventions, while also contributing to administrative tasks, education, and research endeavors. The AAENP supports the utilization of NPs in EMS to the full extent of their licensure, education, and scope of practice based on state and agency regulations.

TRAINING AND QUALIFICATIONS

NPs who work in EMS need specialized training and qualifications, although the specific criteria for this developing sub-specialty are not yet welldefined. It is recommended that NPs who work in EMS pursue national board certification as a family nurse practitioner (FNP), followed by postgraduate certification as an emergency nurse practitioner (ENP). Board certification for FNP is possible after completion of an accredited academic program. ENP certification through the American Academy of Nurse Practitioners Certification Board is available to currently certified FNPs who have met the eligibility options to take the national exam and is further discussed in Chapter 7.1.

Gaining additional clinical experience in the EMS setting would also be advantageous. NPs without any previous prehospital experience or postgraduate training may benefit from enrolling in emergency medical technician (EMT) or paramedic programs, which are offered through community colleges, universities, or some private companies. Completion of the program allows students to sit for the National Registry of EMT or Paramedic exam. This option has been available to nurses interested in flight nursing as a means of providing the necessary training and experience for nurses to work safely in prehospital roles and could easily translate to prehospital NPs. Once a national standard curriculum has been adopted for NPs working in EMS, seeking additional EMS certification may or may not be required moving forward.

Currently, only a few states acknowledge the role of prehospital registered nurses and advanced practice providers in their EMS systems. This lack of recognition means that in many states, there are no specific laws, standards, or legal protections in place to govern the practice of EMS NPs. This situation underscores the need for further attention and advocacy to address the unique challenges faced by EMS NPs in the prehospital care setting.

DIRECT PATIENT CARE

Direct Field Response

NPs working in EMS can be dispatched to 911 calls for emergency medical assistance. They provide on-scene medical services, often in collaboration with other EMS personnel. The EMS NP may respond either as part of a two-person ambulance team or, more commonly, as a secondary responder. Depending on the model and local guidelines, EMS NPs may have varying levels of responsibility, ranging from handling only low-acuity calls to a broader range of acuity levels. Some 911 dispatch centers equipped with triage capabilities may trigger a tiered response that could include an EMS NP. Standing operating procedures can include additional treatment options and procedures for the EMS NP.

Mobile Integrated Healthcare

Mobile integrated healthcare (MIH), also known as community paramedicine, is a model of providing patient-centered and cost-effective medical services outside the hospital setting. MIH programs can be beneficial for patients with mental illness or those with frequent exacerbations of chronic disease, high utilizers of healthcare resources, or those who have transportation or financial barriers to healthcare (Gregg et al., 2019). MIH expands access to healthcare for patients in underserved and remote communities. NPs may collaborate with other healthcare professionals to provide high-quality and coordinated care for these patients (Georgiev et al., 2019). MIH programs aim to reduce healthcare costs, reduce ED visits for non-emergent conditions, prevent hospital readmissions, and improve the management of chronic diseases. Telemedicine expands access to MIH services and allows for virtual consultations with NPs, leading to reductions in unnecessary EMS transports (Gregg et al., 2019). MIH programs continue to evolve addressing other unmet community needs, such as end-of-life and palliative care (Van Vuuren et al., 2021), management of opioid use disorders (Hern et al., 2023), behavioral health, and healthcare navigation.

Street Medicine

Street medicine refers to medical care that is provided to individuals who are experiencing homelessness, living in poverty, or otherwise marginalized and who may not have access to traditional healthcare services (Enich, 2022). NPs deliver care directly on the streets, in shelters, or in other nonclinical settings to meet the patient's unique needs. In this environment, NPs may work collaboratively with physicians, social workers, outreach workers, and other healthcare professionals to provide wrap-around health services and referrals, harm reduction services, psychosocial case management, life necessities, education, and advocacy (Enich, 2022).

Critical Care Transport Teams

Critical care transport teams are tasked with responding to healthcare facilities or directly to scenes to manage patients with critical illnesses or injuries. Their responsibility also includes transporting patients back to tertiary facilities, typically utilizing ambulance or air medical services. The team often consists of specially trained registered nurses, paramedics, respiratory therapists, and/or EMTs. In the past, NPs were primarily utilized on neonatal or pediatric specialty transport teams. However, in recent years, there has been an increased use of NPs on other types of critical care transport teams, including helicopter EMS. Providing critical care services to these populations may require additional acute care academic preparation and specialized training.

Event and Mass Gathering Medical Care

Event medicine focuses on providing medical care and support during large public gatherings or events. These events may include concerts, festivals, sports events, or any other mass gathering of people (Schwartz et al., 2015). The primary goal of event medicine is to ensure the safety and well-being of participants and attendees by providing medical support in the event of an injury or medical emergency. ENPs can collaborate with local agencies and health systems to assess potential risks and develop emergency response plans. ENPs can also provide direct patient care at medical stations and function as an emergency responder to individual or large-scale incidents.

Disaster Medicine

Disaster medicine is a specialty focused on preparedness and response to natural or man-made disasters. ENPs play a vital role in disaster situations and are often included in hospital, local, state, and federal disaster response teams. ENPs work in a range of settings during a disaster, including EMS, mobile medical units, EDs, and field hospitals. During disasters, ENPs may be involved in triaging patients, providing medical treatment and interventions, and coordinating with other healthcare providers. ENPs may collaborate to develop and implement emergency response plans, participate in disaster drills and exercises, and educate the public about disaster preparedness. In some cases, ENPs may have a designated position within the incident command structure.

Austere and Wilderness Medicine

Austere and wilderness medicine involves providing medical care in remote or challenging environments where conventional resources may be limited or unavailable. This specialty encompasses various outdoor physical activities like hiking, camping, and mountaineering and also involves traveling to remote or austere areas such as high altitudes, deserts, jungles, and polar regions. This specialty often demands creative problem-solving to provide medical care in extreme conditions like natural disasters, expeditions, humanitarian crises, military operations, or other scenarios where the medical infrastructure has been disrupted or destroyed. NPs who work in this particular area need specialized skills and training that go beyond traditional academic preparation. This is because they must be able to adjust to the challenges and limitations of the environment and the physical demands of this type of work.

Tactical Medicine

Tactical medicine is a specialized area of prehospital medicine that involves providing immediate medical care in high-risk or tactical situations, such as during law enforcement activities, combat environments, and other high-risk emergency situations. Healthcare in tactical environments ensures that both patients and tactical personnel receive the highest level of care, ultimately bridging the gap between frontline medical response and definitive care facilities. The integration of NPs into tactical medical teams not only enhances the overall medical capacity and effectiveness of these units but also brings an essential occupational health component. NPs can benefit from additional training such as a tactical combat casualty care course and knowledge of local law enforcement protocols.

Public Health

Public health aims to prevent diseases, extend life expectancy, and improve the overall health and welfare of communities. NPs play a crucial role in addressing social determinants of health and promoting community wellness through education, screenings, and timely interventions (Georgiev et al., 2019). Additionally, NPs can contribute to emergency preparedness and response efforts by working collaboratively with public health agencies to plan for and manage potential outbreaks or natural disasters. The COVID-19 pandemic enhanced the relationship between EMS and public health.

Healthcare in the Home

The landscape of healthcare is rapidly changing, driven by advances in technology, telemedicine, remote monitoring capabilities, and the evolving needs of patients. One significant development in recent years is the emergence of healthcare at-home services, which encompasses a range of options such as convenient care, urgent care, and hospital-at-home services. Since the COVID-19 pandemic, there has been a noticeable rise in the availability of these options, as emergency declaration waivers have permitted a greater range of healthcare services to be provided at home. Patients can receive treatment and recover in a familiar environment, leading to enhanced patient satisfaction and improved outcomes. This also alleviates the strain on EDs and reduces healthcare costs. The role of the NP is integral to these services, as they provide expert clinical care and oversight in this new care delivery model (Gaillard & Russinoff, 2023).

Leadership and Administrative Roles

EMS NPs with advanced education in healthcare leadership not only deliver patient care but can also provide administrative support in clinical and operational capacities, alongside the EMS medical director. They develop evidence-based guidelines and protocols for EMS systems, conduct employee training and assessments, and offer medical control to EMS clinicians based on their state's scope of practice. In large-scale incidents, EMS NPs assume leadership roles within the incident command structure and contribute to proactive triage during critical care interfacility transfers. Their expertise as seasoned clinicians proves valuable in case reviews and documentation audits, while their effective collaboration with multidisciplinary teams ensures optimal outcomes. They also contribute to quality assurance and improvement initiatives at various levels and may take on leadership roles or engage in original research to generate novel knowledge in the field (AAENP, 2022; Wright et al., 2021).

THE EMERGENCY TRIAGE, TREAT, AND TRANSPORT MODEL

The ET3 model, or emergency triage, treat, and transport, represents an innovative payment and service delivery approach devised by the Centers for Medicare and Medicaid Services (CMS) in the United States. This model aims to enhance the quality of emergency care while minimizing unnecessary hospital admissions and ED visits. In the ET3 model, ambulance providers can transport patients to alternative destinations like urgent care centers or primary care providers or offer treatment in place by a qualified healthcare provider. NPs can be integral to the ET3 model by offering on-site medical care and/or telehealth services for patients who do not require hospital transport. Currently being piloted in selected regions across the United States, the ET3 model has the potential to reshape the way emergency care is administered (Sorelle, 2019).

EARLY ADOPTERS OF NURSE PRACTITIONERS IN EMERGENCY MEDICAL SERVICES

The Los Angeles Fire Department's advanced provider response unit (APRU) deploys trained NPs to provide on-site medical care in emergency situations, reducing the need for ambulance transport to hospitals. These NPs bring advanced medical training to the field, enabling them to provide prompt evaluation, treatment, and discharge for individuals contacting 911 with non-life-threatening primary or urgent care concerns. They conduct health assessments in the home and assist with chronic disease management for frequent 911 callers. Additionally, the service conducts on-site medical clearance for specific mental health patients, offering the possibility of direct transportation to a psychiatric urgent care facility. The implementation of APRU has required extensive training and coordination within the fire department to ensure NPs can function effectively in emergency services. This initiative has proven to enhance patient care, alleviate strain on emergency services, and showcase the valuable role of NPs in EMS (Sanko et al., 2020)

The Austin-Travis County Emergency Medical Services (ATCEMS) has integrated NPs with paramedic training into its emergency medical response system. The system introduced the role of paramedic practitioner, a term representing both EMS NPs and PAs, who are responsible for diagnosing, treating, and determining patient disposition in the field. Paramedic practitioners not only provide immediate care for a broad range of acute conditions but also serve in various leadership and education roles within the system, while also being an integral part of mobile integrated health teams and other specialty EMS teams. This helps alleviate strain on hospitals and reduces healthcare costs. Paramedic practitioners respond to scene calls as a primary or secondary responder, reducing traditional ambulance deployment costs. By treating and managing various medical conditions on-site, they avoid unnecessary hospital admissions and improve patient care. This innovative approach showcases ATCEMS's commitment to integrating advanced practice roles for more effective and efficient EMS (Austintexas.gov, 2022).

SUMMARY

The evolving role of EMS NPs marks a significant advancement in healthcare delivery and emergency response. The integration of NPs into EMS teams brings forth a unique set of skills, knowledge, and expertise that complements existing capabilities of EMS. NPs are equipped to provide comprehensive and specialized care in the prehospital setting, bridging the gap between traditional EMS providers and hospital-based care. Their ability to assess, diagnose, and initiate appropriate treatments in real time can significantly improve patient outcomes and reduce the burden on EDs. EMS NPs play an important role in community education, preventive care, and disaster response. With the ongoing evolution of the healthcare landscape, the inclusion of EMS NPs as essential members of the emergency response team will transform our approach to prehospital care.

REFERENCES

American Academy of Emergency Nurse Practitioners. (2022, May). *Role of nurse practitioners in emergency medical services: An AAENP position statement*, NP in EMS Role Position Statement_Approved051022. pdf (memberclicks.net)

Austintexas.gov. (2022, March 23). *EMS paramedic practitioners program is expanding to meet needs of the community*, Right Vision Media. https://www.austintexas.gov/news/ems-paramedic-practitioners-program-expanding-meet-needs-community

Enich, M., Tiderington, E., & Ure, A. (2022). Street medicine: A scoping review of program elements. *International Journal on Homelessness, 3*(2), 295–343. https://doi.org/10.5206/ijoh.2022.2.15134

Gaillard, G., & Russinoff, I. (2023). Hospital at home: A change in the course of care. *Journal of the American Association of Nurse Practitioners, 35*(3), 179–182. https://doi.org/10.1097/JXX.0000000000000814

Georgiev, R., Stryckman, B., & Velez, R. (2019). The integral role of nurse practitioners in community paramedicine. *The Journal for Nurse Practitioners, 15*(10), 725–731. https://doi.org/10.1016/j.nurpra.2019.07.019

Gregg, A., Tutek, J., Leatherwood, M. D., Crawford, W., Friend, R., Crowther, M., & McKinney, R. (2019). Systematic review of community paramedicine and EMS mobile integrated health care interventions in the United States. *Population Health Management*, 22(3), 213–222. https://doi.org/10.1089/pop.2018.0 114

Hern, H. G., Lara, V., Goldstein, D., Kalmin, M., Kidane, S., Shoptaw, S., Tzvieli, O., & Herring, A. A. (2023). Prehospital buprenorphine treatment for opioid use disorder by paramedics: First year results of the EMS buprenorphine use pilot. *Prehospital Emergency Care*, 27(3), 334–342. https://doi.org/10.1080/109 03127.2022.2061661

National Association of EMS Physicians. (2023). *About us*. https://naemsp.org/about-us/

Sanko, S., Kashani, S., Ito, T., Guggenheim, A., Fei, S., & Eckstein, M. (2020). Advanced practice providers in the field: Implementation of the Los Angeles Fire Department advanced provider response unit. *Prehospital emergency care*, 24(5), 693–703. https://doi.org/10.1080/10903127.2019.1666199

Schwartz, B., Nafziger, S., Milsten, A., Luk, J., & Yancey, A., 2nd (2015). Mass Gathering Medical Care: Resource Document for the National Association of EMS Physicians Position Statement. *Prehospital Emergency Care*, 19(4), 559–568.

Sorelle, R. (2019). News: ET3 could revolutionize EMS transport. *Emergency Medicine News*, 41(7), 22. https://doi.org/10.1097/01.EEM.0000574780.22839.26

Van Vuuren, J., Thomas, B., Agarwal, G., Macdermott, S., Kinsman, L., O'Meara, P., & Spelten, E. (2021). Reshaping healthcare delivery for elderly patients: The role of community paramedicine; a systematic review. *BMC Health Services Research*, 21(1). https://doi.org/10.1186/s12913-020-06037-0

Wright, D., Baker, T., Muthersbaugh, H., Platt, T., & Kerr. (2021). Position statement: The role of the EMS physician assistant (PA) and nurse practitioner (NP) in EMS systems. *Prehospital Emergency Care*. https://doi.org/10.1080/10903127.2021.1977878

CHAPTER 5.1

Significance of Standards

Dian Dowling Evans
Sue Hoyt

INTRODUCTION

Practice standards and competencies define the provision of competent care and foundations of patient care management for practice and support evaluation of clinician proficiencies by providing measurable outcomes that can be used to assess evolving clinical abilities through the spectrum of novice to expert. The emergency nurse practitioner (ENP) practice standards separate knowledge, tasks, and procedures that are placed under the domains for which the standard is reflected. In many cases, multiple actions can be used to describe the various standards as an ENP progresses in proficiency and the ability to manage more complex patient presentations. A standard will, in many cases, be utilized for building upon a specific task or procedure in the clinical setting, and an action or descriptor term may progress from a basic-knowledge action to a synthesis or performance action.

CHAPTER 5.2

Competencies for the Emergency Nurse Practitioner

David House

INTRODUCTION

In 2008, the first set of competencies for the emergency nurse practitioner (ENP) was developed by a validation work team comprised of experts and validated using the findings from a Delphi study identifying the skills and procedures common to nurse practitioner (NP) practice in emergency care (Davis et al., 2022; Emergency Nurses Association [ENA], 2008). Over the past decade, the role and scope of the ENP has grown rapidly, requiring expertise beyond entry-level competencies. This expanded role and scope of practice led the AAENP in 2018 to publish a new set of competencies based on the American Academy of Nurse Practitioners Certification Board's (AANPCB, 2016) practice analysis of NP practice in emergency care (Davis et al., 2022). Subsequently, the ENA initiated a work group to review, revise, and update the previous 2008 ENP competencies, resulting in the 2019 ENP competencies (ENA, 2019), which were affirmed by the American Nurses Association (ANA) in 2020.

EMERGENCY NURSE PRACTITIONER COMPETENCIES

Variation in these two competencies created confusion, resulting in a call for a unified, single set of ENP competencies. Subject matter experts from both the AAENP and the ENA, using a crosswalk methodology, identified no significant differences between the two documents (Davis et al., 2022). The unified 2021 ENP competencies were aligned with the National Organization of Nurse Practitioner Faculties (NONPF) NP Core Competencies and ensured congruence with *The Essentials: Core Competencies for Professional Nursing Education* (Davis et al., 2022). In 2022, the 2021 emergency nurse competencies were recognized and endorsed by the AAENPs, the ENA, and the NONPF.

Nurse Practitioner Core and Emergency Nurse Practitioner Competency Comparison

Nurse practitioner core competencies for entry to practice were first identified by the NONPF in 1990 (NONPF, 2022). Over time, these competencies evolved due to the transition of NP educational preparation from the master's level to the Doctor of Nursing Practice (DNP) level. In 2017, NONPF updated the previous 2014 NP core competencies to include adult-gerontology acute care and primary care NP competencies, reflecting suggested curriculum content (NONPF, 2017). The most recent revision led to the 2022 NONPF NP role core competencies, which were scaffolded to the 2021 AACN *Essentials*, reflecting the advanced-level nursing education sub-competencies and specialty competencies (NONPF, 2022).

The 2022 NONPF entry-to-practice core competencies are essential behaviors for all NPs, regardless of population focus (NONPF, 2022). ENPs require specialized knowledge, skills, and abilities to provide care across the life span. For entry to practice, the 2021 ENP competencies (see **Table 1**) not only build upon the 2022 NONPF NP core competencies but also complement the 2021 American Nurses Credentialing Center (ANCC) Level 2 sub-competencies for advanced practice specialties. **Table 2** illustrates how the ENP competencies align with the 2022 NONPF competencies and provides exemplars of recommended curriculum content to support the NP core competencies.

TABLE 1: EMERGENCY NURSE PRACTITIONER COMPETENCIES

Domain 1: Medical Screening

1. Performs a medical screening exam for all patients presenting for care
2. Obtains an appropriate history pertinent to the presenting complaint
3. Performs a pertinent, developmentally appropriate physical examination
4. Identifies differential diagnoses requiring immediate intervention
5. Identifies the potential for rapid physiologic and/or mental health deterioration or life-threatening instability
(e.g., suicidal risk, infectious disease/sepsis, shock)
6. Initiates measures to maximize patient safety throughout the emergency care encounter
7. Evaluates assigned triage level for appropriateness based on a medical screening examination

Domain 2: Medical Decision-Making

1. Formulates differential diagnoses to determine emergent versus non-emergent conditions
2. Prioritizes differential diagnoses using advanced clinical reasoning, with consideration of the likelihood for morbidity or mortality
3. Evaluates need for and results of diagnostic testing based on evidence-based recommendations to ensure patient safety
4. Implements clinical decision-making for management plan development

Domain 3: Patient Management

1. Ensures safety of the patient and care team during delivery of emergency care
2. Formulates an individualized, dynamic plan of care to address the stabilization and initial treatment of emergent and non-emergent conditions
3. Provides emergency stabilization of patients experiencing physiologic and/or mental health deterioration or life-threatening instability
4. Prescribes therapies based on current, evidence-based recommendations for emergency care

(continued)

TABLE 1: EMERGENCY NURSE PRACTITIONER COMPETENCIES (*CONTINUED*)

5. Performs diagnostic, procedural, and therapeutic interventions based on current, evidence-based recommendations

6. Reassesses and modifies plan of care based on the dynamic patient condition (change to only one action)

7. Optimizes patient-centered care through interprofessional partnerships and communication

8. Collaborates with patients, families, significant others, and healthcare team to provide safe, effective, and individualized culturally competent care

9. Provides disaster and mass casualty patient management

10. Assesses health literacy in patients and families to promote informed decision-making and optimal participation in care

11. Ensures documentation of patient encounter to ensure safe transitions of patient care

Domain 4: Patient Disposition

1. Develops a plan for safe, effective, and evidence-based disposition plan using shared decision-making with patients and families

2. Implements appropriate patient disposition responsive to demographic trends

3. Communicates patient information effectively to ensure safe transitions in care

4. Selects appropriate intra- and inter-facility patient transport modality

Domain 5: Professional, Legal, and Ethical Practices

1. Incorporates current knowledge and evidence to guide practice and care delivery

2. Manages patient presentation and disposition in accordance with provisions of the EMTALA

3. Provides care in accordance with legal, professional, and ethical responsibilities

4. Actively leads and/or participates in interdisciplinary disaster preparedness and response (change to only one action)

5. Identifies needs of vulnerable populations and intervenes appropriately (change to only one action)

6. Records essential elements of the patient care encounter to facilitate correct coding and billing

7. Integrates culturally competent care into practice

8. Provides family-centered care protective of vulnerable persons and populations across the life span

9. Documents essential elements of patient care in accordance with regulatory and institutional standards

10. Functions as leader, mentor, educator, and/or policy developer to advocate for and ensure delivery of equitable emergency care

11. Contributes to research, quality improvement, and translational science to advance the body of knowledge in emergency care

EMTALA, Emergency Medical Treatment and Active Labor Act; NP, nurse practitioner.

TABLE 2: ALIGNMENT OF EMERGENCY AND CORE COMPETENCIES

NP Domain 1: Knowledge of Nursing Practice
The nurse practitioner integrates, translates, and applies established and evolving scientific knowledge from diverse sources as the basis for ethical clinical judgement, innovation, and diagnostic reasoning.

NP Core Competencies (NONPF, 2022)	Curriculum Content to Support NP Core Competencies (NONPF, 2022)[a]	Emergency NP Competencies	Curriculum Content to Support Emergency NP Competencies[b]
NP 1.1 Demonstrate an understanding of the discipline of nursing's and the NP's role distinct perspective and where shared perspectives exist with other disciplines.	**NP 1.1h**: Integrate historical, foundational, and population-focused knowledge into NP practice. **NP 1.1i**: Translate evidence from nursing science and other sciences into NP practice. **NP 1.1j**: Evaluate the application of nursing science to NP practice.		
NP 1.2 Apply theory and research-based knowledge from nursing, the arts, humanities, and other sciences.	**NP 1.2k**: Synthesize evidence from nursing and other disciplines to inform and improve NP practice at a micro, meso, and macro level. **NP 1.2l**: Translate science-based theories and concepts to guide one's overall NP practice. **NP 1.2m**: Employ ethical decision-making to manage and evaluate patient care and population health. **NP 1.2n**: Practice socially responsible leadership.		
NP 1.3 Demonstrate clinical judgment founded on a broad knowledge base.	**NP 1.3f**: Demonstrate clinical judgment using a systematic approach to inform, improve, and advance NP practice processes and outcomes. **NP 1.3g**: Demonstrate clinical judgement to inform and improve NP practice based on the foundational knowledge of advanced physiology/pathophysiology, advanced health assessment, and advanced pharmacology. **NP 1.3h**: Synthesize current and emerging evidence to influence NP practice.	5.1 Incorporates current knowledge and evidence to guide practice and care delivery	Integration of decision-making tools and evidence-based guidelines into evaluation and management (e.g., HEART score, NEXUS criteria, NIH Stroke Scale) Application of principles of safety related to healthcare processes across the life span within the emergency care environment Methods for translation and integration of research into emergency care Strategies for lifelong learning

[a]Neither required nor comprehensive, this list reflects only suggested content specific to the core competencies.
[b]Neither required nor comprehensive, this list reflects only suggested content specific to the ENP competencies.

(continued)

TABLE 2: ALIGNMENT OF EMERGENCY AND CORE COMPETENCIES (*CONTINUED*)

NP Core Competencies (NONPF, 2022)	Curriculum Content to Support NP Core Competencies (NONPF, 2022)[a]	Emergency NP Competencies	Curriculum Content to Support Emergency NP Competencies[b]
NP Domain 2: Person-Centered Care *The nurse practitioner uses evidence-based and best practices to design, manage, and evaluate comprehensive person-centered care that is within the regulatory and educational scope of practice. Fundamental to person-centered care is respect for diversity, differences, preferences, values, needs, resources, and determinants of health unique to the individual.*			
NP 2.1 Engage with individuals and/or caregivers in establishing a caring relationship.	**NP 2.1f**: Practice holistic person-centered care to include confidentiality, privacy, comfort, emotional support, mutual trust, and respect. **NP 2.1g**: Engage in shared decision-making with consideration of determinants of health.	**3.10** Assesses health literacy in patients and families to promote informed decision-making and optimal participation in care **5.8** Provides family-centered care protective of vulnerable persons and populations across the life span **3.8** Collaborates with patients, families, significant others, and healthcare team to provide safe, effective, and individualized culturally competent care	
NP 2.2 Communicate effectively with individuals.	**NP 2.2k**: Utilize communication tools and techniques to promote therapeutic relationships with individuals and/or caregiver. **NP 2.2l**: Apply motivational interviewing techniques to engage individual and/or caregiver in management of health. **NP 2.2m**: Communicate findings to the interprofessional team, including the preceptor, in a systematic, concise manner to accurately convey the health status of the patient. **NP 2.2n**: Demonstrate empathy and compassion in communication with others.	**4.3** Communicates patient information effectively to ensure safe transitions in care.	

[a]Neither required nor comprehensive, this list reflects only suggested content specific to the core competencies.
[b]Neither required nor comprehensive, this list reflects only suggested content specific to the ENP competencies.

(continued)

TABLE 2: ALIGNMENT OF EMERGENCY AND CORE COMPETENCIES (*CONTINUED*)

NP Core Competencies (NONPF, 2022)	Curriculum Content to Support NP Core Competencies (NONPF, 2022)[a]	Emergency NP Competencies	Curriculum Content to Support Emergency NP Competencies[b]
NP 2.3 Integrate advanced assessment in NP practice.	**NP 2.3i**: Utilize advanced critical thinking to determine the appropriate focused or comprehensive relevant patient history. **NP 2.3j**: Apply advanced assessment skills to perform a comprehensive patient physical assessment utilizing appropriate techniques. **NP 2.3k**: Apply advanced assessment skills to perform a focused patient physical assessment utilizing appropriate techniques. **NP 2.3l**: Order the appropriate diagnostic and screening tests based on patient's risk factors and chief complaint. **NP 2.3m**: Identify health risk factors. **NP 2.3n**: Evaluate determinants of health that may influence the patient's well-being. **NP 2.3o**: Utilize appropriate evidence-based screening tools. **NP 2.3p**: Document comprehensive history, screening, and assessment.	**1.1** Performs a medical screening exam for all patients presenting for care **1.2** Obtains an appropriate history pertinent to the presenting complaint **1.3** Performs a pertinent, developmentally appropriate physical examination **1.7** Evaluates assigned triage level for appropriateness based on a medical screening examination **2.3** Evaluates need for and results of diagnostic testing based on evidence-based recommendations to ensure patient safety	Screening strategies for availability of patient and family social needs/resources Skills to perform diagnostic and therapeutic procedures Risk assessment of physiologic and psychologic conditions which impact care delivery Documentation techniques to support safety and reimbursement Utilization of appropriate resources and technologies to provide and improve healthcare outcomes for patients, including the following: ■ Point-of-care ultrasound ■ Telehealth and telepresence
NP 2.4 Diagnose actual or potential health problems and needs.		**1.4** Identifies differential diagnoses according to chief complaint which require immediate intervention **1.5** Identifies the potential for rapid physiologic and/or mental health deterioration or life-threatening instability (e.g., suicidal risk, infectious disease/sepsis, shock)	

[a]Neither required nor comprehensive, this list reflects only suggested content specific to the core competencies.
[b]Neither required nor comprehensive, this list reflects only suggested content specific to the ENP competencies.

(continued)

TABLE 2: ALIGNMENT OF EMERGENCY AND CORE COMPETENCIES (*CONTINUED*)

NP Core Competencies (NONPF, 2022)	Curriculum Content to Support NP Core Competencies (NONPF, 2022)[a]	Emergency NP Competencies	Curriculum Content to Support Emergency NP Competencies[b]
		2.1 Formulates differential diagnoses to determine emergent versus non-emergent conditions **2.2** Prioritizes differential diagnoses using advanced clinical reasoning, with consideration of the likelihood for morbidity or mortality	
	NP 2.4h: Analyze physical findings to differentiate between normal, variations of normal, and signs of pathology to formulate actual and differential diagnoses.		
	NP 2.4i: Utilize diagnostic reasoning to formulate actual and differential diagnoses.		
NP 2.5 Manage care of individuals.	*NP 2.5k*: Provide holistic person-centered care by developing a mutually acceptable, cost-conscious, and evidence-based plan of care. *NP 2.5l*: Synthesize data to develop and initiate a person-centered plan of care. *NP 2.5m*: Prescribe medications safely and accurately using patient data and following legal and regulatory guidelines.	**2.4** Implements medical decision-making for management plan development **3.2** Formulates an individualized, dynamic plan of care to address the stabilization and initial treatment of emergent and non-emergent conditions	Interpretation of imaging studies Best practices for safe patient management, including pharmacologic, therapeutic, and behavioral interventions

[a]Neither required nor comprehensive, this list reflects only suggested content specific to the core competencies.
[b]Neither required nor comprehensive, this list reflects only suggested content specific to the ENP competencies.

(continued)

TABLE 2: ALIGNMENT OF EMERGENCY AND CORE COMPETENCIES (*CONTINUED*)

NP Core Competencies (NONPF, 2022)	Curriculum Content to Support NP Core Competencies (NONPF, 2022)[a]	Emergency NP Competencies	Curriculum Content to Support Emergency NP Competencies[b]
	NP 2.5n: Order appropriate nonpharmacologic interventions. **NP 2.5o**: Anticipate risks and take action to mitigate adverse events. **NP 2.5p**: Incorporate health promotion, maintenance, and restoration of health into plan of care.	3.3 Provides emergency stabilization of patients experiencing physiologic and/ or mental health deterioration or life-threatening instability 3.4 Prescribes therapies based on current, evidence-based recommendations for emergency care 3.5 Performs diagnostic, procedural, and therapeutic interventions based on current, evidence-based recommendations	
NP 2.6 Demonstrate accountability for care delivery.	**NP 2.6k**: Provide healthcare services within scope of practice boundaries, which include health promotion, disease prevention, anticipatory guidance, counseling, disease management, palliative care, and end-of-life care. **NP 2.6l**: Collaborate with the interprofessional team to formulate a plan of care. **NP 2.6m**: Order consultations or referrals based on evidence and standards of professional care. **NP 2.6n**: Document the comprehensive care provided. **NP 2.6o**: Engage caregivers and support systems in care planning for the individual.		

[a]Neither required nor comprehensive, this list reflects only suggested content specific to the core competencies.
[b]Neither required nor comprehensive, this list reflects only suggested content specific to the ENP competencies.

(*continued*)

TABLE 2: ALIGNMENT OF EMERGENCY AND CORE COMPETENCIES (*CONTINUED*)

NP Core Competencies (NONPF, 2022)	Curriculum Content to Support NP Core Competencies (NONPF, 2022)[a]	Emergency NP Competencies	Curriculum Content to Support Emergency NP Competencies[b]
NP 2.7 Evaluate outcomes of care.	**NP 2.7g**: Evaluate individual outcomes based on evidence-based interventions. **NP 2.7h**: Revise plan of care based on effectiveness. **NP 2.7i**: Analyze data to evaluate interventions, inequities, and gaps in care.	3.6 Reassesses and modifies plan of care based on the dynamic patient condition 4.1 Develops a plan for safe, effective, and evidence-based disposition using shared decision-making with patients and families 4.2 Implements appropriate patient disposition responsive to demographic trends 4.4 Selects appropriate intra- and inter-facility patient transport modality	
NP 2.8 Promote self-care management.	**NP 2.8k**: Integrate the principles of self-care management. **NP 2.8l**: Incorporate coaching in patient and family self-care management. **NP 2.8m**: Create partnerships with community organizations to support self-care management.		
NP 2.9 Provide care coordination.	**NP 2.9k**: Implement evidence-based guidelines and strategies that enable effective transitions of care and care coordination.	4.3 Communicates patient information effectively to ensure safe transitions in care	

NP Domain 3: Population Health
The nurse practitioner partners, across the care continuum, with public health, healthcare systems, community, academic community, governmental, and other entities to integrate foundational NP knowledge into culturally competent practices to increase health promotion and disease prevention strategies in effect the care of populations.

NP 3.1 Manage population health.	**NP 3.1o**: Evaluate outcomes of population health using available sources of data to inform NP practice, guidelines, and policies. **NP 3.1p**: Integrate findings of population health data to impact competent care.		

[a]Neither required nor comprehensive, this list reflects only suggested content specific to the core competencies.
[b]Neither required nor comprehensive, this list reflects only suggested content specific to the ENP competencies.

(continued)

TABLE 2: ALIGNMENT OF EMERGENCY AND CORE COMPETENCIES (*CONTINUED*)

NP Core Competencies (NONPF, 2022)	Curriculum Content to Support NP Core Competencies (NONPF, 2022)[a]	Emergency NP Competencies	Curriculum Content to Support Emergency NP Competencies[b]
NP 3.2 Engage in effective partnerships.	**NP 3.2i**: Contribute clinical expertise and knowledge from advanced practice to interprofessional efforts to protect and improve health.		
NP 3.3 Consider the socioeconomic impact of the delivery of healthcare.	**NP 3.3g**: Appraise ethical, legal, and social factors to guide population health policy development.	**5.5** Identifies needs of vulnerable populations and intervenes appropriately	Strategies to support improving social determinants of health Communication and advocacy strategies to promote the ENP role among policy makers
NP 3.4 Advance equitable population health policy.			Resource utilization to promote ethical policies for access, equity, and quality in emergency care
NP 3.5 Demonstrate advocacy strategies.			
NP 3.6 Advance preparedness to protect population health during disasters and public health emergencies.	**NP 3.6k**: Summarize the unique roles and responsibilities of NPs in emergency preparedness and disaster response. **3.6l**: Collaborate with a team to advance preparedness for potential public health emergencies. **NP 3.6m**: Evaluate the impact of globalization on population health.	**3.9** Provides disaster and mass casualty patient management **5.4** Actively leads and/or participates in interdisciplinary disaster preparedness and response	Mass casualty situations and triage ▪ Implements methods of disaster triage ▪ Provides treatment and resource allocation as applicable ▪ Collaborates with the disaster response team (incident command system) as indicated by institutional policies Emergency preparedness and response ▪ Nuclear/biological/ chemical ▪ Natural disasters ▪ Civil unrest ▪ Mass casualty ▪ Pandemic

NP Domain 4: Practice Scholarship and Translational Science
The nurse practitioner generates, appraises, synthesizes, translates, integrates, and disseminates knowledge to improve person-centered health and systems of care.

[a]Neither required nor comprehensive, this list reflects only suggested content specific to the core competencies.
[b]Neither required nor comprehensive, this list reflects only suggested content specific to the ENP competencies.

(continued)

TABLE 2: ALIGNMENT OF EMERGENCY AND CORE COMPETENCIES (*CONTINUED*)

NP Core Competencies (NONPF, 2022)	Curriculum Content to Support NP Core Competencies (NONPF, 2022)[a]	Emergency NP Competencies	Curriculum Content to Support Emergency NP Competencies[b]
NP 4.1 Advance the scholarship of NP nursing practice.	**NP 4.1n**: Translate advanced practice knowledge to inform practice and patient outcomes. **NP 4.1o**: Lead scholarly activities resulting in the focus of the translation and dissemination of contemporary evidence into practice. **NP 4.1p**: Apply clinical investigative skills to improve health outcomes.	**5.11** Contributes to research, quality improvement, and translational science to advance the body of knowledge in emergency care	Foster awareness of emergency care within the broader complex healthcare systems as the basis for practice inquiry. Translation of nursing knowledge for quality improvement and research which support the evolution and delivery of safe emergency care
NP 4.2 Integrate best evidence into NP practice.	**NP 4.2l**: Evaluate quality improvement processes and evidence-based outcomes. **NP 4.2m**: Disseminate findings from quality improvement, implementation science, and research to improve healthcare delivery and patient outcome.		
NP 4.3 Promote the ethical conduct of scholarly activities.	**NP 4.3j**: Translate knowledge from clinical practice to improve population health outcomes through diversity, equity, and inclusion. **NP 4.3k**: Utilize ethical principles to ensure participant safety through scholarship activities.		
NP Domain 5: Quality and Safety *The nurse practitioner utilizes knowledge and principles of translational and improvement science methodologies to improve quality and safety for providers, patients, populations, and systems of care.*			
NP 5.1 Apply quality improvement principles in care delivery.	**NP 5.1p**: Systematically evaluate quality and outcomes of care using quality improvement principles. **NP 5.1q**: Evaluate the relationships and influence of access, populations, cost, quality, and safety on healthcare.		

[a]Neither required nor comprehensive, this list reflects only suggested content specific to the core competencies.
[b]Neither required nor comprehensive, this list reflects only suggested content specific to the ENP competencies.

(*continued*)

TABLE 2: ALIGNMENT OF EMERGENCY AND CORE COMPETENCIES (*CONTINUED*)

NP Core Competencies (NONPF, 2022)	Curriculum Content to Support NP Core Competencies (NONPF, 2022)[a]	Emergency NP Competencies	Curriculum Content to Support Emergency NP Competencies[b]
	NP 5.1r: Evaluate the impact of organizational systems in healthcare to include care processes, financing, marketing, and policy.		
NP 5.2 Contribute to a culture of patient safety.	*NP 5.2k*: Build a culture of safety through quality improvement methods and evidence-based interventions.	**1.6** Initiates measures to maximize patient safety throughout the emergency care encounter	Innovative delivery models to support patient access to quality and cost-effective care Exemplars of unique risks within emergency care settings Methods for risk reduction and promotion of patient and staff safety, including the following: ■ Fall prevention ■ Verbal de-escalation ■ Work place violence ■ Recognition of human trafficking, exploitation, and abuse Evidence-based practices that promote patient and provider safety in acute and critical care
NP 5.3 Contribute to a culture of provider and work environment safety.		**3.1** Ensures safety of the patient and care team during delivery of emergency care	Strategies to promote the delivery of cost-effective care while maintaining quality and safety Strategies to promote resilience and self-care as an ENP

NP Domain 6: Interprofessional Collaboration in Practice
The nurse practitioner collaborates with the interprofessional team to provide care through meaningful communication and active participation in person-centered and population-centered care.

NP Core Competencies	Curriculum Content to Support NP Core Competencies	Emergency NP Competencies	Curriculum Content to Support Emergency NP Competencies
NP 6.1 Communicate in a manner that facilitates a partnership approach to quality care delivery.	*NP 6.1m*: Engage in collaboration with multiple interprofessional stakeholders (e.g., individuals, community, integrated healthcare teams, and policy makers) to impact a diverse and inclusive healthcare system.	**3.7** Optimizes patient-centered care through interprofessional partnerships and communication **5.7** Integrates culturally competent care into practice	Tools for standardized communication into interactions with other healthcare team members. Leadership skills and interprofessional team dynamics within emergency care and across transitions of care

[a]Neither required nor comprehensive, this list reflects only suggested content specific to the core competencies.
[b]Neither required nor comprehensive, this list reflects only suggested content specific to the ENP competencies.

(continued)

TABLE 2: ALIGNMENT OF EMERGENCY AND CORE COMPETENCIES (*CONTINUED*)

NP Core Competencies (NONPF, 2022)	Curriculum Content to Support NP Core Competencies (NONPF, 2022)[a]	Emergency NP Competencies	Curriculum Content to Support Emergency NP Competencies[b]
	NP 6.1n: Demonstrate equitable and quality healthcare through interprofessional collaboration with the healthcare team. *NP 6.1o*: Advocate for the patient as a member of the healthcare team. *NP 6.1p*: Demonstrate sensitivity to diverse organizations, cultures, and populations.		
NP 6.2 Perform effectively in different team roles, using principles and values of team dynamics.	*NP 6.2k*: Assume different roles (e.g., member, leader) within the interprofessional, healthcare team.		
NP 6.3 Use knowledge of nursing and other professions to address healthcare needs.			
NP 6.4 Work with other professions to maintain a climate of mutual learning, respect, and shared values.	*NP 6.4j*: Promote a climate of respect, dignity, inclusion, integrity, civility, and trust to foster collaboration within the healthcare team. *NP 6.4k*: Collaborate to develop, implement, and evaluate healthcare strategies to optimize safe, effective systems of care.		

NP Domain 7: Health Systems
The nurse practitioner demonstrates organizational and systems leadership to improve healthcare outcome.

NP Core Competencies (NONPF, 2022)	Curriculum Content to Support NP Core Competencies (NONPF, 2022)[a]	Emergency NP Competencies	Curriculum Content to Support Emergency NP Competencies[b]
NP 7.1 Apply knowledge of systems to work effectively across the continuum of care.	*NP 7.1i*: Apply knowledge of organizational practices and complex systems to improve healthcare delivery.		

[a]Neither required nor comprehensive, this list reflects only suggested content specific to the core competencies.
[b]Neither required nor comprehensive, this list reflects only suggested content specific to the ENP competencies.

(continued)

TABLE 2: ALIGNMENT OF EMERGENCY AND CORE COMPETENCIES (*CONTINUED*)

NP Core Competencies (NONPF, 2022)	Curriculum Content to Support NP Core Competencies (NONPF, 2022)[a]	Emergency NP Competencies	Curriculum Content to Support Emergency NP Competencies[b]
NP 7.2 Incorporate consideration of cost-effectiveness of care.	*NP 7.2m*: Demonstrate fiduciary stewardship in the delivery of quality care.	5.6 Records essential elements of the patient care encounter to facilitate correct coding and billing	Strategies to promote the delivery of cost-effective care
NP 7.3 Optimize system effectiveness through application of innovation and evidence-based practice.			
NP Domain 8: Technology and Information Literacy *The nurse practitioner envisions, appraises, and utilizes informatics and healthcare technologies to deliver care.*			
NP 8.1 Appraise the available information and communication technologies used in the care of patients, communities, and populations.	*NP 8.1l*: Evaluate technologies and communication platforms in the care of patients.		
NP 8.2 Use information and communication technologies to gather data, create information, and generate knowledge.	*NP 8.2k*: Analyze data to impact care delivery at the person, population, or systems levels. *NP 8.2l*: Use technology systems to generate, analyze, and interpret data on variables for the evaluation of healthcare. *NP 8.2m*: Select appropriate technology and communication tools to promote engagement and share credible information that is congruent with patient needs, values, and learning styles.		

[a]Neither required nor comprehensive, this list reflects only suggested content specific to the core competencies.
[b]Neither required nor comprehensive, this list reflects only suggested content specific to the ENP competencies.

(*continued*)

TABLE 2: ALIGNMENT OF EMERGENCY AND CORE COMPETENCIES (*CONTINUED*)

NP Core Competencies (NONPF, 2022)	Curriculum Content to Support NP Core Competencies (NONPF, 2022)[a]	Emergency NP Competencies	Curriculum Content to Support Emergency NP Competencies[b]
NP 8.3 Use information and communications technologies and informatics processes to deliver safe care to diverse populations in a variety of settings.		**3.11** Ensures documentation of patient encounter to ensure safe transitions of patient care	Strategies for accurate and timely documentation.
NP 8.4 Use information and communications technology to support documentation of care and communication among providers, patients, and all system levels.	**NP 8.4h**: Assess the patient's and caregiver's learning and communication needs to address gaps in access, knowledge, and information literacy. **NP 8.4i**: Evaluate the design and implementation of clinical information systems within the contexts of quality care, accountability, ethics, and cost-effectiveness.	**3.10** Assesses health literacy in patients and families to promote informed decision-making and optimal participation in care **5.9** Documents essential elements of patient care in accordance with regulatory and institutional standards	Assessment of health literacy of patients and families Incorporation of pertinent patient health records across care continuum congruent with legal and ethical standards Utilization of appropriate resources and technologies to provide and improve healthcare outcomes for patients ▪ Point-of-care ultrasound ▪ Telehealth and telepresence
NP 8.5 Use information and communications technologies in accordance with ethical, legal, professional, and regulatory standards and workplace policies in the delivery of care.	**NP 8.5m**: Use information technology safely, legally, and ethically to manage data to ensure quality care and organizational accountability to promote interprofessional communication.		

NP Domain 9: Professional Acumen
The nurse practitioner demonstrates the attributes and perspectives of the nursing profession and adherence to ethical principles while functioning as a committed equal partner of the interprofessional healthcare team.

[a]Neither required nor comprehensive, this list reflects only suggested content specific to the core competencies.
[b]Neither required nor comprehensive, this list reflects only suggested content specific to the ENP competencies.

(*continued*)

TABLE 2: ALIGNMENT OF EMERGENCY AND CORE COMPETENCIES (*CONTINUED*)

NP Core Competencies (NONPF, 2022)	Curriculum Content to Support NP Core Competencies (NONPF, 2022)[a]	Emergency NP Competencies	Curriculum Content to Support Emergency NP Competencies[b]
NP 9.1 Demonstrate an ethical comportment in one's practice reflective of nursing's mission to society.	**NP 9.1l**: Demonstrate the ability to apply ethical principles in complex health care situations. **NP 9.1m**: Develop strategies to prevent one's own personal biases from interfering with delivery of quality care. **NP 9.1n**: Actively seek opportunities for continuous improvement in professional practice.	**5.3** Provides care in accordance with legal, professional, and ethical responsibilities	Methods for incorporation of inclusivity of ethical, spiritual, and cultural relativism among patients and healthcare teams. Connections between policy and ethical decision-making in emergency care, including the following: ■ Emancipation ■ Advance directives ■ End-of-life care ■ Organ/tissue procurement ■ Informed consent
NP 9.2 Employ participatory approach to NP care.	**NP 9.2m**: Demonstrate an NP professional identity. **NP 9.2n**: Demonstrate accountability to practice within the regulatory standard and scope of educational preparation.		Strategies to support implementation of the full scope of practice ENP role
NP 9.3 Demonstrate accountability to the individual, society, and profession.	**NP 9.3p**: Participate in professional organizations to advance the NP profession and improve health. **NP 9.3q**: Reflect on past experiences to guide present and future practice.		
NP 9.4 Comply with relevant laws, policies, and regulations.	**NP 9.4i**: Advocate for policies that support population focus NPs to practice at the full extent of their education. **NP 9.4j**: Articulate the regulatory process that guides NP practice at the national and individual state level.	**5.2** Manages patient presentation and disposition in accordance with provisions of the EMTALA.	Laws, regulations, and policies which shape and define research and delivery of emergency care (e.g., the EMTALA and reimbursement policies) Transitions in care ■ EMTALA transfers ■ Interprofessional collaboration to ensure state regulations, applicable laws, and institutional policies are followed

[a]Neither required nor comprehensive, this list reflects only suggested content specific to the core competencies.
[b]Neither required nor comprehensive, this list reflects only suggested content specific to the ENP competencies.

(continued)

TABLE 2: ALIGNMENT OF EMERGENCY AND CORE COMPETENCIES (*CONTINUED*)

NP Core Competencies (NONPF, 2022)	Curriculum Content to Support NP Core Competencies (NONPF, 2022)[a]	Emergency NP Competencies	Curriculum Content to Support Emergency NP Competencies[b]
NP 9.5 Demonstrate the professional identity of nursing.	**NP 9.5j**: Articulate the NP's unique professional identity to other interprofessional team members and the public. **NP 9.5k**: Demonstrate the ability to effectively educate and mentor peers, students, or members of the interprofessional healthcare team.		
NP 9.6 Integrate diversity, equity, and inclusion as core to one's professional identity.			
NP Domain 10: Personal and Professional Leadership *The nurse practitioner participates in professional and personal growth activities to develop a sustainable progression toward professional and interpersonal maturity, improved resilience, and robust leadership capacity.*			
NP 10.1 Demonstrate a commitment to personal health and well-being.	**NP 10.1e**: Create an environment that promotes self-care, health, and well-being. **NP 10.1f**: Support for whole-person health and holistic well-being of self.		
NP 10.2 Demonstrate professional maturity.	**NP 10.2**: Demonstrate responsibility to practice in the NP population focus area defined by your education, certification, and license. **NP 10.2l**: Employ empathy to communicate effectively. **NP 10.2m**: Conduct self in a professional manner. **NP 10.2n**: Uphold standards of the NP profession.		
NP 10.3 Develop capacity for leadership.	**NP 10.3r**: Articulate the complex leadership role of the NP. **NP 10.3s**: Execute leadership skills in the translation of new knowledge to improve outcomes.	**5.10** Functions as leader, mentor, educator, and/or policy developer to advocate for and ensure delivery of equitable emergency care	Leadership skills and interprofessional team dynamics within emergency care and across transitions of care

[a]Neither required nor comprehensive, this list reflects only suggested content specific to the core competencies.
[b]Neither required nor comprehensive, this list reflects only suggested content specific to the ENP competencies.

(continued)

TABLE 2: ALIGNMENT OF EMERGENCY AND CORE COMPETENCIES (*CONTINUED*)

NP Core Competencies (NONPF, 2022)	Curriculum Content to Support NP Core Competencies (NONPF, 2022)[a]	Emergency NP Competencies	Curriculum Content to Support Emergency NP Competencies[b]
	NP 10.3t: Provide leadership on teams, and in different team roles, across a variety of practice settings. **NP 10.3u**: Mentor peers. **NP 10.3v**: Engage in advocacy efforts to address health disparities, social justice, and equity to improve healthcare outcomes.		Impact of participation in professional organizations to ■ Influence health policy ■ Promote access to emergency care ■ Advocate for the emergency NP role Strategies to function as change agent and champion

[a]Neither required nor comprehensive, this list reflects only suggested content specific to the core competencies.
[b]Neither required nor comprehensive, this list reflects only suggested content specific to the ENP competencies.
EMTALA, Emergency Medical Treatment and Active Labor Act; ENP, emergency nurse practitioner; HEART, history, ECG, age, risk factors, and troponin levels; NEXUS, National Emergency Radiography Utilization Study; NIH, National Institutes of Health; NP, nurse practitioner.

REFERENCES

American Academy of Nurse Practitioners Certification Board. (2016). *Executive summary of the 2016 practice analysis of emergency nurse practitioners*. Author.

American Association of Colleges of Nursing. (2021). *The essentials: Core competencies for professional nursing education*. https://www.aacnnursing.org/Portals/42/AcademicNursing/pdf/Essentials-2021.pdf

Davis, W., Hallman, M. G., Denke, N., House, D. T., Fuller-Switzer, D., & Wilbeck, J. (2022). A collaboration to unify emergency nurse practitioner competencies. *Journal for Nurse Practitioners, 18*(8), 889–892. https://doi.org/10.1016/j.nurpra.2022.06.014

Emergency Nurses Association. (2008). *Competencies for nurse practitioners in emergency care*. https://www.ena.org/docs/default-source/education-document-library/enpcompetencies_final.pdf?sfvrsn=f75b4634_0

Emergency Nurses Association. (2019). *Emergency nurse practitioner competencies*. https://www.ena.org/docs/default-source/education-document-library/enpcompetencies_final.pdf?sfvrsn=f75b4634_0

National Organization of Nurse Practitioner Faculties. (2022). *National organization of nurse practitioner faculties' nurse practitioner role core competencies*. https://www.nonpf.org/page/14

National Organization of Nurse Practitioner Faculty. (2017). *Nurse practitioner core competencies content*. https://cdn.ymaws.com/www.nonpf.org/resource/resmgr/competencies/20170516_NPCoreCompsContentF.pdf

CHAPTER 5.3

Standards of Practice

Dian Dowling Evans

INTRODUCTION

The emergency nurse practitioner (ENP) role is unique in that it spans population and acuity continuums. Emergency care focuses on potential life-threatening conditions irrespective of the patient's initial chief complaint or reason for seeking care. ENPs must be prepared to provide primary care and acute resuscitation, as well as manage complex, unstable conditions in patients of all ages.

ROLE OF THE EMERGENCY NURSE PRACTITIONER

- ENPs are certified practitioners.
- ENPs provide care to patients in ambulatory, urgent, and emergent care settings.
- ENPs assess, diagnose, and manage episodic illnesses, injuries, and acute exacerbations of chronic diseases.
- ENPs are prepared to manage patients across the life span, within the scope of population-area nurse practitioner (NP) education and national certification, inclusive of acuity levels ranging from nonurgent to urgent and emergent conditions.
- In managing the acute resuscitative stage of emergency care, ENPs engage in patient prioritization, triage, medical decision-making, differential diagnosis, patient management, monitoring, ongoing evaluation, appropriate consultation, and in coordinating the transfer of care.
- ENPs order and interpret diagnostic studies (e.g., labs, imaging) and prescribe pharmacologic and non-pharmacologic therapies.
- ENPs instruct patients, families, and/or significant others with regard to health/wellness along with injury prevention/patient safety.
- ENPs work collaboratively with other healthcare providers, allied/auxiliary healthcare personnel, and stakeholders.
- ENPs are advocates, researchers, consultants, and educators. ENPs are culturally competent.
- ENPs engage in public health emergency preparedness and response efforts.

EMERGENCY NURSE PRACTITIONER ACCOUNTABILITY

- ENP practice is accountable to patients, families, and communities and provides evidence-based quality healthcare based on national standards. ENP practice conforms to professional ethical codes of conduct.
- ENPs meet national certification requirements.
- ENPs undergo peer review and periodic clinical outcome evaluation.
- ENPs provide evidence of emergency continued professional development via continuing education, on-the-job training, or postgraduate-specific fellowships to meet ongoing clinical practice requirements.

EMERGENCY NURSE PRACTITIONER RESPONSIBILITY

- ENPs are responsible to the public as consumers of healthcare and, therefore, keep abreast of the constantly changing landscape of healthcare trends and of the latest evidence-based research.
- ENPs take full responsibility for continued professional development.
- ENPs are leaders who are active in their relevant professional organizations.
- ENPs are actively engaged with health policy initiatives.

EMERGENCY NURSE PRACTITIONER QUALIFICATIONS AND COMPETENCIES

- ENPs possess the necessary clinical competencies to provide optimal care to patients in ambulatory, urgent, and emergent care settings.
- ENP education builds upon NP entry-into-practice knowledge and skills and requires a minimum of a master's-level preparation or specialized preparation at the post-master's or doctoral level.
- ENPs demonstrate competencies by applying standardized care guidelines in their clinical practice. Other ways of maintaining competencies include participation in maintaining continuing education, quality improvement processes, and peer reviews—including the systematic periodic review of records and treatment plans—while maintaining certification in compliance with current laws and regulations.

EMERGENCY NURSE PRACTITIONER PRIORITIZATION OF CARE

- ENPs incorporate evidence-based practice as their framework for managing patient conditions. This process includes the following components: assessment, differential diagnoses/diagnosis, medical decision-making, and treatment/management.

ASSESSMENT

- ENPs assess and triage a patient's condition by obtaining a focused and pertinent history, identifying risk factors, performing an appropriate focused/complete physical examination, and ordering and/or providing preventative or diagnostic procedures.

DIFFERENTIAL DIAGNOSES

■ ENPs develop a differential diagnosis and/or diagnoses of both life-threatening and nonlife-threatening conditions by utilizing critical thinking while simultaneously synthesizing and analyzing patient data. ENPs establish differential diagnoses based on the patient's medical history, physical exam findings, and interpretation of diagnostic studies, while continually establishing priorities to meet the needs of the patient, their family, and/or the community.

MEDICAL DECISION-MAKING

■ ENPs utilize critical thinking during medical screenings and diagnostic processes by synthesizing and analyzing the data (i.e., all known diagnoses being treated; undiagnosed conditions being evaluated; treatments implemented, considered, or planned) to execute a plan of care including stabilization, resuscitation of unstable conditions, and the transfer of care when appropriate.

■ ENPs provide medical screening evaluations in accordance with the Emergency Medical Treatment and Active Labor Act (EMTALA). This includes documentation of the chief complaint and pertinent history, incorporating health risk factors and physical exam findings; interpretation of diagnostic data, including the rationale for the medical necessity of tests; and medical decision-making with differential diagnoses, adding ongoing evaluation of patient progress and response to treatment to determine the plan of care.

TREATMENT/MANAGEMENT

■ ENPs provide individualized, cost-effective, evidence-based plans of care to maximize a patient's well-being. ENPs' plan of care consists of ordering/ interpreting diagnostics, ordering/performing therapeutic interventions including non-pharmacologic therapies, prescribing pharmacologic agents, developing patient-specific education plans, and making timely referrals/ consultations as needed. ENPs also provide acute resuscitation and stabilization of life-threatening conditions and coordinate transfers to critical care providers/ facilities as warranted.

■ Plan implementation: ENP interventions include established priorities of care that are individualized and based on current evidence-based guidelines.

■ Follow-up and evaluation: ENPs determine the effectiveness of a patient's treatment plan by following a systematic process including documentation of patient care outcomes, ongoing reassessment, and/or plan modification to optimize a patient's health status within the context of emergency care.

■ An ENP's practice emphasizes health education including the provision of community resources for patients and their families.

■ Facilitation of patient self-care: ENPs facilitate entry into the healthcare system and provide competent care in a safe environment. ENPs promote patient participation by providing the necessary information to promote optimal health and make informed health decisions. The ENP consults with other healthcare personnel as needed and appropriately utilizes healthcare resources.

EMERGENCY NURSE PRACTITIONER DOCUMENTATION

- ENPs document accurately, legibly, and in a timely manner while maintaining confidential emergency care medical records.

EMERGENCY NURSE PRACTITIONER INTERPROFESSIONAL/ COLLABORATIVE RESPONSIBILITIES

- ENPs participate as interprofessional/collaborative members in emergency care, interacting with colleagues to promote comprehensive, quality patient care.

EMERGENCY NURSE PRACTITIONER PATIENT ADVOCATE RESPONSIBILITIES

- Ethical and legal standards provide the basis of patient advocacy. As an advocate, ENPs participate in health policy regulatory and legislative activities. ENPs are able to define their role to patients, families, and other professionals.

PRACTICE-BASED RESEARCH

- ENPs promote research by formulating clinical inquiries, by conducting or participating in research and quality improvement studies, and by disseminating and incorporating findings into their clinical practice.

OTHER ROLES

- ENPs blend the roles of clinician, mentor, educator, researcher, leader, interdisciplinary team member, and consultant.

EMERGENCY NURSE PRACTITIONER PROCEDURES ACROSS THE LIFE SPAN

Beyond the technical ability to perform a procedure, knowledge of the context in which procedures may be safely performed is crucial in the provision of emergency care. The practice standards for the ENP, therefore, represent the integration of knowledge, psychomotor ability, and discernment of the need to perform procedures within emergency care settings in collaboration with the healthcare team. Procedures in this specialty span from simple laceration repair to life-saving procedures. Practice analysis data ultimately identified procedures frequently performed by ENPs within 15 specific procedural areas (PSI, 2021).

Table 1 lists the procedures identified during the practice analysis pertinent to ENP practice. While this is not an exhaustive list of the skills identified during the practice analysis, those included represent procedures identified as being applicable across broad clinical settings. Many of the included procedures were not performed frequently yet represent necessary knowledge and are thus included due to the high risk of harm if there is a failure in recognizing the need for the procedure. Differences in state regulations, provider credentialing, and collaborative practice at individual facilities as well as practice settings (e.g., critical access, academic, or tertiary care) will ultimately determine which skills an ENP may perform.

TABLE 1: ENP SKILLS AND PROCEDURES EXAMPLES

PROCEDURAL AREA/ SYSTEM	EXEMPLAR SKILLS AND PROCEDURES
Airway techniques	■ Intubation airway adjuncts ■ Surgical airway ■ Mechanical ventilation ■ Noninvasive ventilatory management ■ Ventilatory monitoring
Resuscitation	■ Cardiopulmonary resuscitation (life span) ■ Post-resuscitative care ■ Blood, fluid, and component therapy ■ Arterial catheter insertion ■ Central venous access (ultrasound guided) ■ Intraosseous infusion ■ Defibrillation
Anesthesia and acute pain management	■ Local anesthesia ■ Regional nerve block ■ Procedural sedation and analgesia
Gastrointestinal	■ Anoscopy ■ Excision of thrombosed hemorrhoid ■ Gastrostomy tube replacement ■ Esophageal/gastric balloon tamponade ■ Paracentesis
Cardiovascular and thoracic	■ Cardiac pacing ■ Cardioversion ■ ECG interpretation ■ Pericardiocentesis ■ Thoracentesis ■ Needle/tube thoracostomy
Cutaneous	■ Escharotomy ■ Incision and drainage ■ Trephination, subungual ■ Wound closure techniques
Head, ear, eye, nose, and throat	■ Control of epistaxis ■ Drainage of peritonsillar abscess ■ Laryngoscopy ■ Lateral canthotomy ■ Slit lamp examination ■ Tonometry ■ Tooth stabilization ■ Corneal foreign body removal ■ Drainage of hematoma (auricular, septal)

(continued)

TABLE 1: ENP SKILLS AND PROCEDURES EXAMPLES (*CONTINUED*)

PROCEDURAL AREA/ SYSTEM	EXEMPLAR SKILLS AND PROCEDURES
Musculoskeletal	■ Arthrocentesis ■ Compartment pressure measurement, fracture/dislocation immobilization techniques, fracture/dislocation reduction techniques ■ Spine immobilization techniques ■ Fasciotomy
Nervous system	■ Lumbar puncture
Obstetrics and gynecology	■ Pelvic examination ■ Precipitous delivery (including complications) ■ Sexual assault examination ■ Bartholin cyst incision and drainage
Renal and urogenital	■ Suprapubic catheter ■ Testicular detorsion
Other diagnostic and therapeutic procedures	■ Foreign body removal ■ Collection and handling of forensic material ■ Point-of-care ultrasound ■ Interpretation of diagnostic imaging (e.g., ultrasound, MRI, CT, radiographs)

ENP, emergency nurse practitioner.

REFERENCE

PSI. (2021). *Practice analysis report: Emergency nurse practitioner.* https://www.aanpcert.org/resource/documents/AANPCB%202021%20ENP%20Practice%20Analysis%20Executive%20Summary.pdf

CHAPTER 6.1

Curricular Essentials Within Academic Emergency Nurse Practitioner Programs

Jennifer Wilbeck

INTRODUCTION

Over the past decade, the creation of new emergency nurse practitioner (ENP) academic programs has accelerated and expanded. This program growth reflects the growing need for nurse practitioners (NPs) entering the emergency workforce and the recognition that emergency-specific competencies in resuscitation, procedural skills, prioritization of care, and complex medical decision-making are essential to the role. Additionally, academic program growth accelerated following the creation of an ENP specialty certification examination by the American Academy of Nurse Practitioners Certification Board (AANPCB) in 2017.

Within U.S. EDs, almost 80% utilize NPs and physician assistants (PAs) to provide care (Wu & Darracq, 2021). Among this advanced practice provider workforce, the NP presence within emergency care has grown and evolved in recent years (Mafi et al., 2022). While the care provided by NPs and PAs may look similar at the bedside (Wu & Darracq, 2021), the educational preparation does not.

ALIGNMENT WITH THE APRN CONSENSUS MODEL

Unlike the educational training of physicians and PAs, NP practice is based on a specific population from the outset of education. As academic programs preparing NPs for practice is targeted toward specific ages and acuities, an initial challenge to ENP education was the alignment of emergency care expertise within an existing population as defined in 2008 by the *Consensus Model for APRN Regulation: Licensure, Accreditation, Certification, and Education* (Consensus Model; APRN Consensus Work Group and National Council of State Boards of Nursing APRN Advisory Committee, 2008). **Figure 1** illustrates the four APRN roles and six population foci. An NP may also specialize in providing care to a more discrete area of their population foci, such as palliative care, oncology, or emergency care.

Ensuring ENP education remains congruent with educational models set forth by the Consensus Model while operating within the confines of state regulatory bodies has proven challenging. As academic NP programs align educational curricular development with specific NP populations delineated by the Consensus Model the selection of the most appropriate population for ENP education was difficult given the variety of care delivery models and practice environments. In 1994, UT Houston began offering the first ENP program preparing graduates for acute care certification.

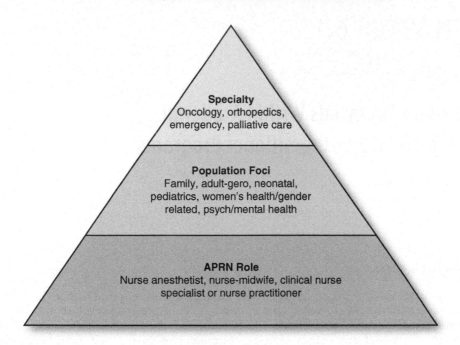

FIGURE 1: APRN roles and population foci as defined by the Consensus Model for APRN Regulation.

Several other programs followed an acute care focus; however, the evolution of healthcare delivery and increasing use of the ED for nonurgent problems necessitated that ENP educational preparation become rooted in primary care, pediatrics, and women's health content.

In more recent years, the acuity of patients seen in the ED, as well as the diversity of ages and acuities, has accelerated. Despite this, the largest percentage of patients encountered in emergency care settings are treated and released and do not require hospitalization or resuscitative care (Emergency Department Benchmarking Alliance, 2017; Rui & Kang, 2014). Given that most emergency care is delivered in settings managing patients across the life span, the family population of NP practice was determined to be the most appropriate foundation for specialty emergency NP education.

Recognizing the different pathways in NP education and the subsequent wide variability in NP readiness to practice in EDs, the American College of Emergency Physicians (ACEP) endorsed ENP specialty education and board certification as an appropriate mechanism to support the preparation of NPs to ensure competent care within emergency care settings (Greene, 2018). Content areas for ENP program curricula were initially proposed in 2017, following the publication of the national ENP practice analysis data (Wilbeck et al., 2017). With the release of updated ENP competencies in 2021 (American Academy of Emergency Nurse Practitioners [AAENP] and Emergency Nurses Association [ENA]), ENP curricular content areas may now be more clearly delineated.

According to the Consensus Model, specialty nursing organizations are charged with providing oversight for their respective specialties (National Council of State Boards of Nursing [NCSBN], 2008). For NPs providing emergency care, that oversight rests with the AAENP. To ensure that programs are consistently providing the educational content to support the unique knowledge, skills, and abilities required for the safe provision of care in emergency settings, the AAENP has established a validation process (see Chapter 6.2, "Validation of Academic Emergency Nurse Practitioner Programs") for curricular evaluation of ENP programs.

EMERGENCY NURSE PRACTITIONER CURRICULAR ESSENTIALS

While academic ENP programs are not individually accredited, programs are evaluated within the context of their population-accredited programs and institutions and should therefore meet all applicable accreditation standards. Accreditation standards for academic schools of nursing, such as those set forth by the National Task Force (NTF) on Quality Nurse Practitioner Education (2022), the Commission on Collegiate Nursing Education (CCNE), and the Accreditation Commission for Education in Nursing (ACEN), guide curricular design. Essential knowledge for inclusion in academic ENP programs thus incorporates competency-based educational standards, the American Association of Colleges of Nursing (AACN) *Essentials* (2021), National Organization of Nurse Practitioner Faculties (NONPF) Core Competencies (2017), and the ENP Competencies (AAENP and ENA Emergency Nurse Practitioner Competencies Work Group, 2021).

Knowledge, Skills, and Abilities in Emergency Care Across the Life Span

Academic programs must provide ENP students with the didactic and clinical knowledge required to manage patients "requiring advanced diagnostic reasoning, risk stratification, and medical decision-making that is distinct from other APRN practices . . . across the lifespan incorporating the trajectory of acuities in the context of the patient's developmental stage" (AAENP and ENA Emergency Nurse Practitioner Competencies Work Group, 2021, p. 7). Comprehensive ENP curricula should therefore encompass the ENP scopes, standards, and competencies. Programs designed in this manner support ENP-specific knowledge, domains, and competencies to prepare graduates for national ENP practice and certification.

Didactic Content

Guided by national role delineation study data, established competencies, and best practices in education, emergency-specific educational curricula have been proposed (Wilbeck et al., 2018; Wilbeck et al., 2017). With increasing momentum for the Doctor of Nursing Practice (DNP) degree as entry to practice, the use of the advanced-level *Essentials* (AACN, 2021) should also be considered during stages of ENP curriculum development and revision. Academic ENP programs must provide students to enter the modern healthcare workforce with competence that spans ages and undifferentiated presentations of varied acuities.

The complexities of providing comprehensive emergency NP education require thoughtful planning of curricular content and sequencing. To ensure student attainment of comprehensive emergency care knowledge, skills, and abilities, ENP program curricular mapping may be used to demonstrate the connectedness of ENP competencies with the program's expectations for student learning and student learning with program activities (Wilbeck et al., 2020). Utilizing identified ENP domains and skills as the organizational framework of this mapping tool, content within specific courses can be identified within the context of the overall academic ENP program sequencing.

Skills and Procedural Content

Common skills and procedures performed by NPs within emergency care settings were identified in the most recent national ENP practice analysis (PSI, 2021) and have been collated into seminal texts available to support academic programs (Campo & Lafferty, 2022; Holleran & Campo, 2022). Table 1 in Chapter 5.3 lists these commonly performed skills and procedures. In the setting of competency-based education, faculty must not only provide the didactic knowledge to identify the need for and ability to safely perform procedures but also to assess student progression toward competence in procedural skills.

Competency Assessment

While a certain threshold of clinical hours within academic programs is required to demonstrate competency and ultimately obtain certification, the AAENP validation program of academic programs (described in Chapter 6.2) focuses on competency-based outcomes rather than a standard number of clinical hours. Evaluation of student progression toward attainment of core competencies may involve diverse assessments over time. These may include case studies and/or reflective analysis, formative and summative simulation experiences, objective structured clinical examinations (OSCEs) using standardized patients, and demonstrated performance of procedural skills (Battista et al., 2018; Hege et al., 2018; Wilbeck et al., 2020).

The progression toward clinical competence may also be assessed using entrustable professional activities (EPAs) and milestones as objective measures for assessing progressive proficiency in competency development (Beeson et al., 2014; Hoyt et al., 2017). Utilized with graduate medical education, the activities described as EPAs typically encompass multiple discrete competencies. For example, an EPA might include the sub-competencies of medical decision-making, history taking, and performing an appropriate physical examination. The EPA is the collective global competency comprised of these subcompetencies that is observable and measurable and can be used to demonstrate a learner's overall ability to practice safely and independently (Hart et al., 2019). As a measure of the learner's professional acumen or critical thinking ability, an EPA can track a learner's progression in professional development over time. Within ENP educational programs, EPAs can incorporate specific skills and procedures (such as patient assessment and central line insertion) as well as targeted competencies. Repeated assessments over time can demonstrate student attainment of both the Time 1 and Time 2 competencies as outlined in the *Essentials*, as well as provide the opportunity to assess ENP-specific competencies.

TYPES OF ACADEMIC PROGRAMS

With the continued evolution of the ENP role and workforce needs, opportunities for academic programs and degrees are expanding. Current options for academic ENP preparation include a Master of Science in Nursing (MSN), post-master's certificate, and DNP programs of study. Recently, the number of students seeking post-master's or doctoral education in emergency care is increasing.

For practicing NPs with certifications in population foci other than family across the life span, most validated academic programs offer mechanisms for post-master's plans of study to support the expansion of educational preparation and scope of practice. Guidelines for gap analyses and individual programs of study must be developed to provide nontraditional students with streamlined educational offerings to meet their individual needs. Given the breadth, diversity, and depth of knowledge required for ENP practice, the DNP option is an appropriate entry to practice preparation in the current workforce landscape. Graduates of all ENP programs, regardless of entry and exit type, must demonstrate attainment of the ENP competencies.

CONCLUSION

Recent projections are that NPs and PAs will provide roughly 20% of emergency care in the coming years (Marco et al., 2021). With increased growth in academic programs offering emergency NP education, delineating and incorporating fundamental content is essential to ensure curricula are robust, targeted, and congruent with applicable competencies. The existing and growing number of resources supporting ENP education provides both the foundation and support for the growth of this unique healthcare workforce role.

REFERENCES

American Academy of Emergency Nurse Practitioners and Emergency Nurses Association Emergency Nurse Practitioner Competencies Work Group. (2021). *Emergency nurse practitioner competencies.* https://aaenp.memberclicks.net/assets/docs/ENPcompetencies_FINAL2.pdf

American Association of Colleges of Nursing. (2021). *The essentials: Core competencies for professional nursing education.* https://www.aacnnursing.org/Portals/42/AcademicNursing/pdf/Essentials-2021.pdf

APRN Consensus Work Group and National Council of State Boards of Nursing APRN Advisory Committee. (2008). *Consensus model for APRN regulation: Licensure, accreditation, certification, and education.* https://www.ncsbn.org/Consensus_Model_for_APRN_Regulation_July_2008.pdf

Battista, A., Konopasky, A., Ramani, D., Ohmer, M., Mikita, J., Howle, A., Krajnik, S., Torre, D., & Durning, S. (2018). Clinical reasoning in the primary care setting: Two scenario-based simulations for residents and attendings. *MedEdPORTAL, 14,* 10773. https://doi.org/10.15766/mep_2374-8265.10773

Beeson, M. S., Warrington, S., Bradford-Saffles, A., & Hart, D. (2014). Entrustable professional activities: Making sense of the emergency medicine milestones. *Journal of Emergency Medicine, 47,* 441–452.

Campo, T. M., & Lafferty, K. A. (2022). *Essential procedures for emergency, urgent, & primary care settings: A clinical companion* (3rd ed.). Springer Publishing.

Emergency Department Benchmarking Alliance. (2017). *Emergency medicine emergency department performance measures, Final Report 2016.* Issued Nov 14, 2017. The Emergency Department Benchmarking Alliance

Greene, J. (2018). New emergency nurse practitioner certification rolled out: Certification offers nurse practitioners head start in emergency department practice. *Annals of Emergency Medicine, 72*(6), 16A–18A. https://doi.org/10.1016/j.annemergmed.2018.10.027

Hart, D., Franzen, D., Beeson, M., Bhat, R., Kulkarni, M., Thibodeau, L., Weizberg, M., & Promes, S. (2019). Integration of entrustable professional activities with the milestones for emergency medicine residents. *The Western Journal of Emergency Medicine, 20*(1), 35–42. https://doi-10.5811/westjem.2018.11.38912

Hege, A., Kononowicz, A., Berman, N., Lenzer, B., & Kiesewetter, J. (2018). Advanced clinical reasoning in virtual patients-development and application of a conceptual framework. *GMS Journal for Medical Education, 35*(1), 1–19. https://www.researchgate.net/publication/321229025_Advancing_clinical_reasoning_in_virtual_patients_-_development_and_application_of_a_conceptual_framework

Holleran, R. S., & Campo, T. M. (2022). *Emergency nurse practitioner core curriculum.* Springer Publishing.

Hoyt, K. S., Ramirez, E., & Proehl, J. A. (2017). Making a case for entrustable professional activities for nurse practitioners in emergency care. *Advanced Emergency of Nursing Journal, 39,* 77–80.

Mafi, J. N., Chen, A., Guo, R., Choi, K., Smulowitz, P., Tseng, C.-H., Ladapo, J. A., & Landon, B. E. (2022). US emergency care patterns among nurse practitioners and physician assistants compared with physicians: a cross-sectional analysis. *BMJ Open, 12*(4), e055138. https://doi.org/10.1136/bmjopen-2021-055138

Marco, C. A., Courtney, D. M., Ling, L. J., Salsberg, E., Reisdorff, E. J., Gallahue, F. E., Suter, R. E., Muelleman, R., Chappell, B., Evans, D. D., Vafaie, N., & Richwine, C. (2021). The emergency medicine physician workforce: Projections for 2030. *Annals of Emergency Medicine, 78*(6), 726–737. https://doi.org/10.1016/j.annemergmed.2021.05.029

National Council of State Boards of Nursing. (2008). *Consensus model for APRN regulation: Licensure, accreditation, certification, & education.* https://www.ncsbn.org/Consensus_Model_for_APRN_Regulation_J uly_2008.pdf

PSI. (2021). Practice analysis report: Emergency nurse practitioner. https://www.aanpcert.org/resource/d ocuments/AANPCB%202021%20ENP%20Practice%20Analysis%20Executive%20Summary.pdf

Rui, P., & Kang, K. (2014). National hospital ambulatory medical care survey: 2014 emergency department summary tables. https://www.cdc.gov/nchs/data/nhamcs/web_tables/2014_ed_web_tables.pdf

Wilbeck, J., Evans, D., Hoyt, K.S., Schumann, L., Ramirez, E., Tyler, D., & Agan, D. (2018). Proposed standardized educational preparation for the emergency nurse practitioner. *Journal of the American Association of Nurse Practitioners, 30*(10), 579–585. https://doi.org/10.1097/JXX.0000000000000133

Wilbeck, J., Evans, D., Hummer, K., & Staebler, S. (2020). Supporting program rigor in newly developed academic programs. *Journal of the American Association of Nurse Practitioners, 32*, 579–582.

Wilbeck, J., Roberts, E., & Rudy, S. (2017). Emergency nurse practitioner core educational content. *Advanced Emergency Nursing Journal, 39*(2), 141–151.

Wu, F., & Darracq, M. A. (2021). Comparing physician assistant and nurse practitioner practice in U.S. emergency departments, 2010-2017. *Western Journal of Emergency Medicine, 22*(5), 1150–1155.

CHAPTER 6.2

Validation of Academic Emergency Nurse Practitioner Programs

Wesley D. Davis
Melanie Gibbons Hallman

INTRODUCTION

The American Academy of Emergency Nurse Practitioners (AAENP) represents nurse practitioners (NPs) caring for the emergency patient population. The *Consensus Model for APRN Regulation: Licensure, Accreditation, Certification, and Education* (APRN Consensus Work Group, National Council of State Boards of Nursing APRN Advisory Committee, 2008) states, "advanced practice registered nurse (APRN) specialties are developed, recognized, and monitored by the profession." Additionally, regulatory bodies, such as state boards of nursing, and national accreditors of nursing programs do not review, regulate, or accredit APRN specialty academic programs; there was not previously a mechanism to ensure quality emergency nurse practitioner (ENP) education.

To ensure quality education and enhance the ENP profession, the AAENP has created validation standards for ENP programs (Davis et al., 2020; Davis et al., 2023). Unlike the regulations for APRN specialties by state boards of nursing and national accreditors of nursing programs, the AAENP's standards focus on providing a strong foundation of programmatic structures and curriculum content, along with requirements for ENP competency and program leadership.

DEFINITION OF VALIDATION

Validation is the official recognition on the AAENP website of an ENP academic program which meets the standards established by the AAENP Validation Committee for the inclusion of appropriate specialty content.

VALIDATION COMMITTEE

The Validation Committee is a standing committee of AAENP that serves as the primary review body for ENP programs applying for initial or continuing validation. Panels of evaluators, who may or may not be members of the Validation Committee, are enlisted to complete the review process. Evaluators are selected and approved by the members of the Validation Committee. Evaluators utilize the *Criteria for Evaluation of Emergency Nurse Practitioner Programs* for the evaluation process **(Table 1)**.

According to the *Criteria for Evaluation of Nurse Practitioner Programs*, "In addition to preparation for national certification in the role and at least one population-focused

---

TABLE 1: CRITERIA FOR EVALUATION OF EMERGENCY NURSE PRACTITIONER ACADEMIC PROGRAMS

EVALUATOR:	DATE OF EVALUATION:
Evaluator area of expertise: ■ Nurse practitioner with academic program design experience ■ ENP practicing in an emergency care setting ■ ENP academic program director/ coordinator/faculty	Evaluator recommendation: ■ Approve ■ Approve with minor revisions ■ Major revisions required

ENP, emergency nurse practitioner.

---

area of practice, programs may prepare students to practice in a specialty or more limited area of practice. Preparation in a specialty *must have additional didactic and clinical hours beyond those required for preparing graduates in the NP role and one population-focused area* [emphasis added]" (National Task Force on Quality Nurse Practitioner Education, 2016). The purpose of the AAENP Validation Committee is to *evaluate the curriculum* that is in addition to the population foci criteria (National Task Force on Quality Nurse Practitioner Education, 2016, 2022) and that prepares the NP for the ENP specialty. As the specialty organization for ENPs, validation of ENP academic programs by AAENP is required to meet the education criteria for the American Academy of Nurse Practitioners Certification Board (AANPCB) certification exam.

AAENP is not an accrediting agency and does not evaluate nursing degree programs. While the Validation Committee coordinates the program review process, ENP academic and clinical experts from across the country complete a double-blinded review of ENP programs.

ACADEMIC PROGRAM EVALUATORS

The AAENP relies on a large network of national ENP experts to evaluate ENP academic programs. The evaluation team will consist of five reviewers as follows:

■ Two ENPs practicing in an emergency care setting, one of which is a clinical preceptor
  ■ The ENP practicing in an emergency care setting serving on the review team either (a) works full time in emergency care as an ENP and has at least 5 years of full-time experience in the role or (b) has worked full time as an ENP for a minimum of 10 years and maintains currency in practice by providing emergency care at least 500 hours per year. The practicing ENP has general knowledge about advanced practice nursing and specialty knowledge in advanced emergency care. The ENP holds current certification as an ENP by AANPCB.
■ Two ENP academic program director/coordinator/faculty
  ■ The ENP faculty member who serves on the review team has expert proficiency in advanced emergency nursing and has demonstrated excellence in NP specialty education and program development. They assist the review team to understand the nature of specialty NP education and the importance of preparing safe and effective ENPs. The ENP academic program director/coordinator/faculty assists the committee in evaluating the ENP academic curricula and faculty roles and qualifications. The ENP director/coordinator/faculty will hold current ENP certification as an ENP by AANPCB.

- One NP with academic program design experience (is not required to be an ENP or work in emergency care)
  - The NP with academic program design experience who serves on the review team has expert proficiency in one or more areas of advanced nursing practice and has expert knowledge of nursing education and program design. They are responsible for assisting the review team to recognize and understand the application of sound pedagogy within the academic program design. Academic program design experts assist the review committee in evaluating ENP academic curricula, evaluative processes, and faculty roles and qualifications.

Procedural Overview

The AAENP Validation Committee has developed a systematic process to assess and evaluate ENP programs to determine alignment with published ENP educational standards. The following documents will inform the process:

- American Academy of Emergency Nurse Practitioners (2016). *Scope and Standards for Emergency Nurse Practitioner Practice*. https://www.aaenp-natl.org/assets/docs/aaenp_scope_and_standards.pdf
- American Academy of Emergency Nurse Practitioners and Emergency Nurses Association Emergency Nurse Practitioner Competencies Work Group. (2021). Emergency nurse practitioner competencies. https://aaenp.memberclicks.net/assets/docs/ENPcompetencies_FINAL2.pdf
- American Academy of Nurse Practitioners Certification Board. (2023). *Emergency nurse practitioner specialty certification: ENP certification handbook*. https://www.aanpcert.org/resource/documents/Emergency%20NP%20Handbook.pdf

A master's degree, postgraduate certificate, or Doctor of Nursing Practice ENP program may request a review by the Validation Committee. The review process is voluntary and is initiated by the institution. The validation procedure consists of the following steps:

1. The program submits an intent for validation review letter using the electronic portal available on the AAENP website. When the letter of intent is received, the Validation Committee will begin recruiting reviewers for the proposed program.
2. The program submits a complete application **(Table 2)** to AAENP requesting a formal review of the ENP program within 6 months of submitting the intent for validation review letter.
   a. It is highly encouraged that the program completes a self-study to assess for deficiencies prior to requesting a formal review. Further details for this process are outlined in the materials provided by AAENP upon submission of the intent for validation review.
   b. It is the university's responsibility to ensure that all identifying information has been removed from the required documentation (except for the director's curriculum vitae (CV) and evidence of certification). The AAENP will not review the material for identifying information prior to distribution to reviewers.
3. Once the application is received, the committee chairperson will perform an initial review of the program information to ensure a complete application has been received. At this point, the timeline for the review process begins (see **Figure 1**).
4. The committee chairperson will review the ENP program director's CV and evidence of certification since this information cannot be de-identified for the reviewers.
5. An evaluation team is appointed by the Validation Committee chairperson to assess the program and determine program alignment with ENP academic

program standards. Each evaluator will complete a report for the Validation Committee within 28 days.

6. In a review of the evaluators' reports, the Validation Committee will determine the validation status of the program (see outcomes in the "Validation Categories" section on p. 83).

7. The Validation Committee chairperson will issue a formal decision letter to the university.

To remain a validated program, the evaluation process must be completed every 5 years.

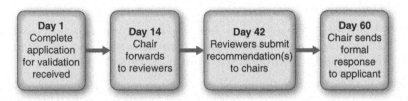

FIGURE 1: Timeline for the validation review process.

TABLE 2: CRITERIA FOR EVALUATION OF EMERGENCY NURSE PRACTITIONER ACADEMIC PROGRAMS

CRITERIA	EVALUATIVE ELEMENT(S)	REQUIRED EVIDENCE	EVALUATOR OBSERVATIONS	ALL ELEMENTS PRESENT (Y/N)
GENERAL REQUIREMENTS				
1.1	The director/coordinator of the ENP program holds current certification as an ENP by AANPCB and has the responsibility of overall leadership for the ENP program. This criterion is reviewed by the Validation Committee chairperson since the required evidence cannot be de-identified.	Curricula vitae, proof of ENP certification by AANPCB, and a statement describing the program director/coordinator's responsibilities to the program		
1.2	All ENP program faculty who teach within the program/track maintain current certification as an ENP by AANPCB. This criterion is reviewed by the Validation Committee chairperson since the required evidence cannot be de-identified.	Curricula vitae and proof of ENP certification by AANPCB		

(continued)

TABLE 2: CRITERIA FOR EVALUATION OF EMERGENCY NURSE PRACTITIONER ACADEMIC PROGRAMS (*CONTINUED*)

CRITERIA	EVALUATIVE ELEMENT(S)	REQUIRED EVIDENCE	EVALUATOR OBSERVATIONS	ALL ELEMENTS PRESENT (Y/N)
1.3	All faculty teaching in the ENP program maintain currency in clinical practice.	A copy of institutional policies or guidelines that support/document the ENP faculty's ability to practice or documentation of faculty practice plan or arrangements		
1.4	The ENP program prepares graduates to meet educational eligibility requirements for ENP certification exam.	Written statement provided to students identifying the ENP certification examination for which they are prepared to meet educational eligibility requirements to apply upon successful completion of the program Documentation demonstrating that the program prepares graduates to meet educational eligibility requirements for the ENP certification exam offered by AANPCB		
1.5	Official program documentation states the ENP specialty focus of educational preparation.	Official documentation (e.g., transcripts or official letters with institutional seal) states the ENP specialty focus of educational preparation		
1.6	The curriculum plan demonstrates appropriate course sequencing.	The curriculum plan documents the course sequencing and prerequisites designed to promote development of competencies. Clinical experiences are supported by preceding or concurrent didactic content.		

(*continued*)

TABLE 2: CRITERIA FOR EVALUATION OF EMERGENCY NURSE PRACTITIONER ACADEMIC PROGRAMS (*CONTINUED*)

CRITERIA	EVALUATIVE ELEMENT(S)	REQUIRED EVIDENCE	EVALUATOR OBSERVATIONS	ALL ELEMENTS PRESENT (Y/N)
1.7	The ENP specialty program/track has a minimum of 300 supervised direct patient care clinical hours dedicated solely to emergency care. These hours must be separate and distinct from any other required clinical hours used to complete other tracks of study. Clinical hours are distributed to support specialty competency development and to allow application of content in a variety of emergency care settings (e.g., in a DNP program, the program of study must clearly articulate which clinical hours are used to meet the DNP requirements and which clinical hours are used to meet the ENP requirements).	The program of study for the graduate and/or postgraduate (full and parttime) including courses, course sequence, number of credit hours, and number of clinical hours per course, as appropriate A brief overview, including course description and objectives for each course, identifying where nationally recognized specialty competencies are included		
1.8	In addition to preparation in the FNP population-focused area of practice, programs may prepare students to practice in the ENP specialty area of practice. Preparation in a specialty must have additional didactic and clinical hours beyond those required for preparing graduates in the FNP role. The clinical hours required to complete the ENP component of the program must be separate and distinct from any other required clinical hours used to complete the FNP component of the program.	The program of study for the graduate and/or postgraduate (full and parttime) including courses, course sequence, number of credit hours, and number of clinical hours per course, as appropriate A brief overview, including course description and objectives for each course, identifying where nationally recognized graduate core, APRN core, and NP role/ population-focused educational standards and core competencies are included		

(*continued*)

TABLE 2: CRITERIA FOR EVALUATION OF EMERGENCY NURSE PRACTITIONER ACADEMIC PROGRAMS (*CONTINUED*)

CRITERIA	EVALUATIVE ELEMENT(S)	REQUIRED EVIDENCE	EVALUATOR OBSERVATIONS	ALL ELEMENTS PRESENT (Y/N)
		A brief overview, including course description and objectives for each course, identifying where nationally recognized specialty competencies are included		
EMERGENCY CARE SKILLS AND PROCEDURES				
2.1	Airway techniques ■ Intubation ■ Airway adjuncts ■ Surgical airways ■ Mechanical ventilation ■ Noninvasive ventilator management ■ Ventilator monitoring	Student handbook, course syllabi, or other appropriate documentation that shows each of the listed skills and procedures are taught by an appropriate simulation[a] modality[b] and are taught across the life span where appropriate. The university/college ENP-prepared faculty must lead the simulation[a] experience and assess student competency in the skills and procedures.		
2.2	Resuscitation ■ Cardiopulmonary resuscitation ■ Neonatal resuscitation ■ Pediatric resuscitation ■ Post-resuscitative care ■ Blood, fluid, and component therapy ■ Arterial catheter insertion ■ Central venous access ■ Intraosseous access ■ Defibrillation	Student handbook, course syllabi, or other appropriate documentation that shows each of the listed skills and procedures are taught by an appropriate simulation[a] modality[b] and are taught across the life span where appropriate. The university/college ENP-prepared faculty must lead the simulation[a] experience and assess student competency in the skills and procedures.		

(continued)

TABLE 2: CRITERIA FOR EVALUATION OF EMERGENCY NURSE PRACTITIONER ACADEMIC PROGRAMS (*CONTINUED*)

CRITERIA	EVALUATIVE ELEMENT(S)	REQUIRED EVIDENCE	EVALUATOR OBSERVATIONS	ALL ELEMENTS PRESENT (Y/N)
2.3	Anesthesia and acute pain management ■ Local anesthesia ■ Regional nerve block ■ Procedural sedation and analgesia	Student handbook, course syllabi, or other appropriate documentation that shows each of the listed skills and procedures are taught by an appropriate simulation[a] modality[b] and are taught across the life span where appropriate. The university/college ENP-prepared faculty must lead the simulation[a] experience and assess student competency in the skills and procedures.		
2.4	Diagnostic and therapeutic procedures: Abdominal and GI ■ Anoscopy ■ Excision of thrombosed hemorrhoid ■ Gastrostomy tube replacement ■ Esophageal/gastric balloon tamponade (e.g., Minnesota/Blakemore/Linton tube) ■ Paracentesis	Student handbook, course syllabi, or other appropriate documentation that shows each of the listed skills and procedures are taught by an appropriate simulation[a] modality[b] and are taught across the life span where appropriate. The university/college ENP-prepared faculty must lead the simulation[a] experience and assess student competency in the skills and procedures.		
2.5	Cardiovascular and thoracic ■ Cardiac pacing ■ Cardioversion ■ ECG interpretation ■ Pericardiocentesis ■ Thoracentesis ■ Needle and tube thoracostomy	Student handbook, course syllabi, or other appropriate documentation that shows each of the listed skills and procedures are taught by an appropriate simulation[a] modality[b]		

(*continued*)

TABLE 2: CRITERIA FOR EVALUATION OF EMERGENCY NURSE PRACTITIONER ACADEMIC PROGRAMS (*CONTINUED*)

CRITERIA	EVALUATIVE ELEMENT(S)	REQUIRED EVIDENCE	EVALUATOR OBSERVATIONS	ALL ELEMENTS PRESENT (Y/N)
		and are taught across the life span where appropriate. The university/college ENP-prepared faculty must lead the simulation[a] experience and assess student competency in the skills and procedures.		
2.6	Cutaneous ■ Escharotomy ■ Incision and drainage ■ Trephination, subungual ■ Wound closure techniques	Student handbook, course syllabi, or other appropriate documentation that shows each of the listed skills and procedures are taught by an appropriate simulation[a] modality[b] and are taught across the life span where appropriate. The university/college ENP-prepared faculty must lead the simulation[a] experience and assess student competency in the skills and procedures.		
2.7	Head, ear, eye, nose, and throat ■ Control of epistaxis ■ Drainage of peritonsillar abscess ■ Laryngoscopy ■ Lateral canthotomy ■ Slit lamp examination ■ Tonometry ■ Tooth stabilization ■ Corneal foreign body removal ■ Drainage of hematoma (auricular, septal)	Student handbook, course syllabi, or other appropriate documentation that shows each of the listed skills and procedures are taught by an appropriate simulation[a] modality[b] and are taught across the life span where appropriate. The university/college ENP-prepared faculty must lead the simulation[a] experience and assess student competency in the skills and procedures.		

(continued)

TABLE 2: CRITERIA FOR EVALUATION OF EMERGENCY NURSE PRACTITIONER ACADEMIC PROGRAMS (*CONTINUED*)

CRITERIA	EVALUATIVE ELEMENT(S)	REQUIRED EVIDENCE	EVALUATOR OBSERVATIONS	ALL ELEMENTS PRESENT (Y/N)
2.8	Musculoskeletal ■ Arthrocentesis ■ Compartment pressure measurement ■ Fracture/dislocation immobilization techniques ■ Fracture/dislocation reduction techniques ■ Spine immobilization techniques ■ Fasciotomy	Student handbook, course syllabi, or other appropriate documentation that shows each of the listed skills and procedures are taught by an appropriate simulation[a] modality[b] and are taught across the life span where appropriate. The university/college ENP-prepared faculty must lead the simulation[a] experience and assess student competency in the skills and procedures.		
2.9	Nervous system ■ Lumbar puncture	Student handbook, course syllabi, or other appropriate documentation that shows each of the listed skills and procedures are taught by an appropriate simulation[a] modality[b] and are taught across the life span where appropriate. The university/college ENP-prepared faculty must lead the simulation[a] experience and assess student competency in the skills and procedures.		
2.10	Obstetrics and gynecology ■ Pelvic examination ■ Precipitous delivery (including complications) ■ Perimortem C-section ■ Sexual assault examination ■ Bartholin cyst incision and drainage	Student handbook, course syllabi, or other appropriate documentation that shows each of the listed skills and procedures are taught by an appropriate simulation[a] modality[b] and are taught across		

(*continued*)

TABLE 2: CRITERIA FOR EVALUATION OF EMERGENCY NURSE PRACTITIONER ACADEMIC PROGRAMS (*CONTINUED*)

CRITERIA	EVALUATIVE ELEMENT(S)	REQUIRED EVIDENCE	EVALUATOR OBSERVATIONS	ALL ELEMENTS PRESENT (Y/N)
		the life span where appropriate. The university/college ENP-prepared faculty must lead the simulation[a] experience and assess student competency in the skills and procedures.		
2.11	Psychobehavioral ▪ Psychiatric screening examination/medical stabilization ▪ Violent patient management/restraint	Student handbook, course syllabi, or other appropriate documentation that shows each of the listed skills and procedures are taught by an appropriate simulation[a] modality[b] and are taught across the life span where appropriate. The university/college ENP-prepared faculty must lead the simulation[a] experience and assess student competency in the skills and procedures.		
2.12	Renal and urogenital ▪ Suprapubic catheter ▪ Testicular detorsion	Student handbook, course syllabi, or other appropriate documentation that shows each of the listed skills and procedures are taught by an appropriate simulation[a] modality[b] and are taught across the life span where appropriate. The university/college ENP-prepared faculty must lead the simulation[a] experience and assess student competency in the skills and procedures.		

(continued)

TABLE 2: CRITERIA FOR EVALUATION OF EMERGENCY NURSE PRACTITIONER ACADEMIC PROGRAMS (*CONTINUED*)

CRITERIA	EVALUATIVE ELEMENT(S)	REQUIRED EVIDENCE	EVALUATOR OBSERVATIONS	ALL ELEMENTS PRESENT (Y/N)
2.13	Other diagnostic and therapeutic procedures ■ Foreign body removal ■ Collection and handling of forensic evidence ■ Point-of-care ultrasound ■ Interpretation of diagnostic imaging (e.g., ultrasound, MRI, CT, radiographs)	Student handbook, course syllabi, or other appropriate documentation that shows each of the listed skills and procedures are taught by an appropriate simulation[a] modality[b] and are taught across the life span where appropriate. The university/college ENP-prepared faculty must lead the simulation[a] experience and assess student competency in the skills and procedures.		

PRACTICE DOMAINS AND COMPETENCIES

3.1	Domain 01: Medical screening ■ Performs a medical screening exam for all patients presenting for care ■ Obtains an appropriate history pertinent to the presenting complaint ■ Performs a pertinent, developmentally appropriate physical examination ■ Identifies differential diagnoses requiring immediate intervention ■ Identifies potential for rapid physiologic and/or mental health deterioration or life-threatening instability (e.g., suicidal risk, infectious disease/sepsis, shock) ■ Evaluates assigned triage level for appropriateness based on a medical screening exam	Course syllabi, assignments, or other appropriate documentation that shows each of the listed domain elements are taught by an appropriate methodology		

(continued)

TABLE 2: CRITERIA FOR EVALUATION OF EMERGENCY NURSE PRACTITIONER ACADEMIC PROGRAMS (*CONTINUED*)

CRITERIA	EVALUATIVE ELEMENT(S)	REQUIRED EVIDENCE	EVALUATOR OBSERVATIONS	ALL ELEMENTS PRESENT (Y/N)
3.2	Domain 02: Medical decision-making ■ Formulates differential diagnoses to determine emergent versus non-emergent conditions ■ Prioritizes differential diagnoses using advanced clinical reasoning, with consideration of the likelihood for morbidity or mortality ■ Evaluates need for and results of diagnostic testing based on evidence-based recommendations to ensure patient safety ■ Implements medical decision-making for management plan development	Course syllabi, assignments, or other appropriate documentation that shows each of the listed domain elements are taught by an appropriate methodology		
3.3	Domain 03: Patient management ■ Ensures safety of the patient and care team during delivery of emergency care ■ Formulates an individualized, dynamic plan of care to address the stabilization and initial treatment of emergent and non-emergent conditions ■ Provides emergency stabilization of patients experiencing physiologic and/or mental health deterioration or life-threatening instability ■ Prescribes therapies based on current, evidence-based recommendations for emergency care	Course syllabi, assignments, or other appropriate documentation that shows each of the listed domain elements are taught by an appropriate methodology		

(continued)

TABLE 2: CRITERIA FOR EVALUATION OF EMERGENCY NURSE PRACTITIONER ACADEMIC PROGRAMS (*CONTINUED*)

CRITERIA	EVALUATIVE ELEMENT(S)	REQUIRED EVIDENCE	EVALUATOR OBSERVATIONS	ALL ELEMENTS PRESENT (Y/N)
	■ Performs diagnostic, procedural, and therapeutic interventions based on current, evidence-based recommendations ■ Reassesses and modifies plan of care based on the dynamic patient condition ■ Optimizes patient-centered care through interprofessional partnerships and communication ■ Collaborates with patients, families, significant others, and the healthcare team to provide safe, effective, and individualized culturally competent care ■ Provides disaster and mass casualty patient management ■ Assesses health literacy in patients and families to promote informed decision-making and optimal participation in care ■ Ensures documentation of patient encounter to ensure safe transitions of patient care			
3.4	Domain 04: Patient disposition ■ Develops a plan for safe, effective, and evidence-based disposition plan using shared decision-making with patients and families ■ Implements appropriate patient disposition responsive to demographic trends	Course syllabi, assignments, or other appropriate documentation that shows each of the listed domain elements are taught by an appropriate methodology		

(continued)

TABLE 2: CRITERIA FOR EVALUATION OF EMERGENCY NURSE PRACTITIONER ACADEMIC PROGRAMS (*CONTINUED*)

CRITERIA	EVALUATIVE ELEMENT(S)	REQUIRED EVIDENCE	EVALUATOR OBSERVATIONS	ALL ELEMENTS PRESENT (Y/N)
	■ Communicates patient information effectively to ensure safe transitions of care ■ Selects appropriate intra- and inter-facility patient transport modality			
3.5	Domain 05: Professional, legal, and ethical practices ■ Incorporates current knowledge and evidence to guide practice care delivery ■ Manages patient presentation and disposition in accordance with provisions of the EMTALA ■ Provides care in accordance with legal, professional, and ethical responsibilities ■ Actively leads and/or participates in interdisciplinary disaster preparedness and response ■ Identifies needs of vulnerable populations and intervenes appropriately ■ Records essential elements of the patient care encounter to facilitate correct coding and billing ■ Integrates culturally competent care into practice ■ Provides family-centered care protective of vulnerable persons and populations across the life span	Course syllabi, assignments, or other appropriate documentation that shows each of the listed domain elements are taught by an appropriate methodology		

(*continued*)

TABLE 2: CRITERIA FOR EVALUATION OF EMERGENCY NURSE PRACTITIONER ACADEMIC PROGRAMS (*CONTINUED*)

CRITERIA	EVALUATIVE ELEMENT(S)	REQUIRED EVIDENCE	EVALUATOR OBSERVATIONS	ALL ELEMENTS PRESENT (Y/N)
	■ Documents essential elements of patient care in accordance with regulatory and institutional standards ■ Functions as a leader, mentor, educator, and/or policy developer to advocate for and ensure delivery of equitable emergency care ■ Contributes to research, quality improvement, and translational science to advance the body of knowledge in emergency care			
PATIENT CONDITIONS				
4.1	General ■ Clinical decision-making tools ■ EMTALA ■ Organ donation ■ Pain control/procedural sedation ■ Palliative care considerations ■ SIRS/sepsis/shock continuums	Course syllabi, assignments, or other appropriate documentation that shows each of the listed elements are taught by an appropriate methodology, to include life-span applications where appropriate		
4.2	Cardiovascular ■ ACS, including STEMI management ■ Antiarrhythmic pharmacology ■ Endocarditis ■ Heart blocks ■ Hypertensive emergencies ■ Myocardial and pericardial disease ■ Vasopressor therapy	Course syllabi, assignments, or other appropriate documentation that shows each of the listed elements are taught by an appropriate methodology, to include life-span applications where appropriate		
4.3	Endocrinology ■ Cholinergic crisis ■ Diabetic ketoacidosis ■ Thyroid storm	Course syllabi, assignments, or other appropriate documentation		

(continued)

TABLE 2: CRITERIA FOR EVALUATION OF EMERGENCY NURSE PRACTITIONER ACADEMIC PROGRAMS (*CONTINUED*)

CRITERIA	EVALUATIVE ELEMENT(S)	REQUIRED EVIDENCE	EVALUATOR OBSERVATIONS	ALL ELEMENTS PRESENT (Y/N)
		that shows each of the listed elements are taught by an appropriate methodology, to include life-span applications where appropriate		
4.4	Environmental ■ Aquatic injuries ■ Hyperthermia/heat stroke ■ Hypothermia ■ Near drowning/ drowning ■ Snake bites	Course syllabi, assignments, or other appropriate documentation that shows each of the listed elements are taught by an appropriate methodology, to include life-span applications where appropriate		
4.5	Gastrointestinal ■ Abdominal compartment syndrome ■ Appendicitis ■ Bowel obstruction ■ Bowel perforation ■ Choledocholithiasis ■ Diverticulitis ■ Foreign bodies ■ Gastrointestinal bleeds ■ Intussusception ■ Mesenteric ischemia ■ Pancreatitis	Course syllabi, assignments, or other appropriate documentation that shows each of the listed elements are taught by an appropriate methodology, to include life-span applications where appropriate		
4.6	Head, ear, eye, nose, and throat ■ Dental emergencies ■ Facial and ocular trauma ■ Post-tonsillectomy bleeding	Course syllabi, assignments, or other appropriate documentation that shows each of the listed elements are taught by an appropriate methodology, to include life-span applications where appropriate		

(continued)

TABLE 2: CRITERIA FOR EVALUATION OF EMERGENCY NURSE PRACTITIONER ACADEMIC PROGRAMS (*CONTINUED*)

CRITERIA	EVALUATIVE ELEMENT(S)	REQUIRED EVIDENCE	EVALUATOR OBSERVATIONS	ALL ELEMENTS PRESENT (Y/N)
4.7	Hematology ■ Acute leukemias ■ Anticoagulation ■ Bleeding diathesis/ blood component therapy ■ Implications of blood and marrow transplant ■ Management of sickle cell crisis/disease ■ Mass transfusion protocols	Course syllabi, assignments, or other appropriate documentation that shows each of the listed elements are taught by an appropriate methodology, to include life-span applications where appropriate		
4.8	Immunology ■ Anaphylaxis	Course syllabi, assignments, or other appropriate documentation that shows each of the listed elements are taught by an appropriate methodology, to include life-span applications where appropriate		
4.9	Infectious disease ■ Fever of unknown origin ■ Infestations ■ Influenza ■ Kawasaki disease ■ Rickettsial and mosquito-borne disease ■ Travel and tropical diseases ■ Tuberculosis	Course syllabi, assignments, or other appropriate documentation that shows each of the listed elements are taught by an appropriate methodology, to include life-span applications where appropriate		
4.10	Integumentary/ dermatology ■ Burn management ■ Life-threatening rashes ■ Wound management	Course syllabi, assignments, or other appropriate documentation that shows each of the listed elements are taught by an appropriate methodology, to include life-span applications where appropriate		

(continued)

TABLE 2: CRITERIA FOR EVALUATION OF EMERGENCY NURSE PRACTITIONER ACADEMIC PROGRAMS (*CONTINUED*)

CRITERIA	EVALUATIVE ELEMENT(S)	REQUIRED EVIDENCE	EVALUATOR OBSERVATIONS	ALL ELEMENTS PRESENT (Y/N)
4.11	Orthopedics/trauma ■ Blunt and penetrating trauma ■ Cauda equina ■ Fracture management ■ Low back pain ■ Multisystem trauma ■ NEXUS criteria ■ Soft-tissue and deep-space infections ■ Traction	Course syllabi, assignments, or other appropriate documentation that shows each of the listed elements are taught by an appropriate methodology, to include life-span applications where appropriate		
4.12	Neurological ■ Closed head injury ■ CVA/TIA ■ Diabetes insipidus and SIADH ■ Evaluation of acute altered mental status ■ Headache ■ Hydrocephalus ■ Meningitis ■ Neuromuscular diseases ■ Peripheral neuropathies ■ Seizures ■ Spinal cord injuries ■ Traumatic brain injuries	Course syllabi, assignments, or other appropriate documentation that shows each of the listed elements are taught by an appropriate methodology, to include life-span applications where appropriate		
4.13	Oncology ■ Graft versus host disease ■ Neutropenic fever ■ Superior vena cava syndrome ■ Tumor lysis syndrome	Course syllabi, assignments, or other appropriate documentation that shows each of the listed elements are taught by an appropriate methodology, to include life-span applications where appropriate		
4.14	Psychiatric ■ Acute psychoses ■ Management of aggressive behavior ■ Suicidal/homicidal ideations ■ Psychiatric medications—acute complications	Course syllabi, assignments, or other appropriate documentation that shows each of the listed elements are taught by an appropriate methodology, to include life-span applications where appropriate		

(continued)

TABLE 2: CRITERIA FOR EVALUATION OF EMERGENCY NURSE PRACTITIONER ACADEMIC PROGRAMS (*CONTINUED*)

CRITERIA	EVALUATIVE ELEMENT(S)	REQUIRED EVIDENCE	EVALUATOR OBSERVATIONS	ALL ELEMENTS PRESENT (Y/N)
4.15	Pulmonary ■ ABG interpretation ■ Acute respiratory failure ■ Foreign bodies/ aspirations ■ Interstitial processes ■ Upper versus lower airway diseases	Course syllabi, assignments, or other appropriate documentation that shows each of the listed elements are taught by an appropriate methodology, to include life-span applications where appropriate		
4.16	Renal ■ Acid–base imbalances ■ Acute kidney injury ■ Alterations in osmolality and electrolytes ■ Emergent dialysis indications ■ PD peritonitis ■ Rhabdomyolysis	Course syllabi, assignments, or other appropriate documentation that shows each of the listed elements are taught by an appropriate methodology, to include life-span applications where appropriate		
4.17	Reproductive ■ GYN surgical emergencies—TOA, ruptured ectopic ■ Preeclampsia/ eclampsia management ■ STI management ■ Threatened/ spontaneous abortions	Course syllabi, assignments, or other appropriate documentation that shows each of the listed elements are taught by an appropriate methodology, to include life-span applications where appropriate		
4.18	Toxicology ■ Anticholinergic crisis management ■ Illicit street drugs/ synthetics ■ Management of alcohol withdrawal ■ Reversal agents ■ Toxidromes/toxic ingestions	Course syllabi, assignments, or other appropriate documentation that shows each of the listed elements are taught by an appropriate methodology, to include life-span applications where appropriate		

(continued)

TABLE 2: CRITERIA FOR EVALUATION OF EMERGENCY NURSE PRACTITIONER ACADEMIC PROGRAMS (*CONTINUED*)

CRITERIA	EVALUATIVE ELEMENT(S)	REQUIRED EVIDENCE	EVALUATOR OBSERVATIONS	ALL ELEMENTS PRESENT (Y/N)
4.19	Urology ■ Acute urinary retention ■ Lithiasis ■ Prostatitis ■ Urethritis ■ UTI/pyelonephritis	Course syllabi, assignments, or other appropriate documentation that shows each of the listed elements are taught by an appropriate methodology, to include life-span applications where appropriate		

Note: Details of the evaluator descriptions and recommendations can be found in the ENP Academic Program Handbook.
[a]Simulation: An educational strategy in which a particular set of conditions are created or replicated to resemble authentic situations that are possible in real life. Simulation can incorporate one or more modalities to promote, improve, or validate a participant's performance (International Nursing Association for Clinical Simulation and Learning, 2016).
[b]Modality: A term used to refer to the type(s) of simulation being used as part of the simulation activity, for example, task trainers, manikin based, standardized/simulated patients, computer based, virtual reality, and hybrid (International Nursing Association for Clinical Simulation and Learning, 2016).
AANPCB, American Academy of Nurse Practitioners Certification Board; ABG, arterial blood gas; ACS, acute coronary syndrome; CVA, cerebral vascular accident; DNP, Doctor of Nursing Practice; EMTALA, Emergency Medical Treatment and Active Labor Act; ENP, emergency nurse practitioner; FNP, family nurse practitioner; GYN, gynecology; NEXUS, National Emergency Radiography Utilization Study; PD, peritoneal dialysis; SIADH, syndrome of inappropriate secretion of antidiuretic hormone; SIRS, systemic inflammatory response syndrome; STEMI, ST-elevation myocardial infarction; STI, sexually transmitted infection; TIA, transient ischemic attack; TOA, tubo-ovarian abscess; UTI, urinary tract infection.

VALIDATION CATEGORIES

Validation

Validation is the recognition status granted by the AAENP Validation Committee to an ENP program that meets the standards set by AAENP.

Validation Pending Minor Revisions

Validation pending minor revisions is assigned to applications that require few or minor revisions to the proposed program. Revised applications are not sent back to the reviewers. The Validation Committee chairperson will review the revised application to ensure that the program has corrected all the deficiencies that were identified in the initial review. Failure to correct all deficiencies will result in validation being denied.

Validation Pending Major Revisions

Validation pending major revisions is assigned to applications that require major revisions. Revised applications will be sent back to the reviewers to ensure that the program has corrected all the deficiencies that were identified in the initial review. Failure to correct all deficiencies will result in validation being denied.

Validation Denied

Validation is denied by AAENP when an ENP program seeking validation does not meet the standards set by AAENP after one revision attempt. Programs denied validation must submit a new application and pay another application fee to begin the review process again.

VALIDATION TERM

The program's validation remains valid for 5 years from the date of the formal decision letter issued by the Validation Committee chairperson. Validation automatically lapses at the conclusion of the 5 years. The AAENP does not grant extensions of validation terms. For validation renewal, there are two options:

1. Submit an application for validation.
   a. The AAENP recommends that programs submit an application for continued validation at least 6 months prior to the program's validation expiration date. For a review of continued validation by the AAENP, the program must submit an application for review.
2. Submit a program self-study for validation.
   a. The self-study option must be elected by submitting a request for self-study on the AAENP website.
   b. The self-study must be submitted to the AAENP Validation Committee before validation expiration.
   c. The self-study must be completed by the ENP program director.
   d. Deficiencies must be accompanied by an action plan to correct the deficiency within 90 days.

PROGRAM CHANGE NOTIFICATION

Validated ENP programs are expected to maintain compliance with the current AAENP standards for program evaluation and maintenance for validation, including advising the AAENP Validation Committee in the event of a change affecting the program. ENP programs that are validated by the AAENP are required to notify the AAENP Validation Committee of any change(s) impacting the ENP program. Changes considered to be significant in nature are closely aligned with what constitutes a substantive change for nursing program accrediting bodies, such as the Commission on Collegiate Nursing Education (2019). For the purposes of ENP validation, significant changes include but are not limited to the following (Commission on Collegiate Nursing Education, 2019):

- change in ownership or oversight of the institution or program, including acquisition by or a merger with another institution;
- a significant reduction in resources of the ENP program such that previously described learning and/or assessment methods are no longer utilized and/or available;
- change in status with a state board of nursing, accrediting or regulatory body, including cases in which the ENP program is placed on warning or probationary status;
- change (including addition, suspension, or closing) in ENP-related degree offerings or program options;
- the addition of courses that represent a significant change in method or location of delivery from those offered when AAENP last evaluated the program

- change in the ENP program director or significant change of faculty composition and size;
- major curricular revisions; and
- ENP-C certification pass rates for all test takers (first time and repeat) less than 80% over a 3-year period.

The letter describing the significant change must be submitted to the AAENP Validation Committee using the electronic portal available on the AAENP website no earlier than 90 days prior to change implementation or occurrence but no later than 90 days after implementation or occurrence of the change. Details for content to be addressed in the letter, including the anticipated implications of the change, are included on the letter template. Once received, the significant change report is reviewed by the AAENP Validation Committee. Upon review of the report, the committee may act to approve the change or may request additional information. Changes in program leadership or other program details reflected on the AAENP website will be updated following receipt of the change notification.

Continued program validation is contingent upon the ENP program director or appropriate university/college official notifying the AAENP Validation Committee of substantive changes in a timely manner. Failure to do so within the time frame noted earlier may result in a loss of program validation.

REFERENCES

American Academy of Emergency Nurse Practitioners. (2016). *Scope and standards for emergency nurse practitioner practice.* https://www.aaenp-natl.org/assets/docs/aaenp_scope_and_standards.pdf

American Academy of Emergency Nurse Practitioners and Emergency Nurses Association Emergency Nurse Practitioner Competencies Work Group. (2021). *Emergency nurse practitioner competencies.* https://aaenp.memberclicks.net/assets/docs/ENPcompetencies_FINAL2.pdf

American Academy of Nurse Practitioners Certification Board. (2023). *Emergency nurse practitioner specialty certification: ENP certification handbook.* https://www.aanpcert.org/resource/documents/Emergency%20NP%20Handbook.pdf

APRN Consensus Work Group, National Council of State Boards of Nursing APRN Advisory Committee. (2008). *Consensus model for APRN regulation: Licensure, accreditation, certification and education.* https://ncsbn.org/Consensus_Model_for_APRN_ Regulation_July_2008.pdf

Commission on Collegiate Nursing Education. (2019). *Procedures for accreditation of baccalaureate and graduate nursing programs.* https://www.aacnnursing.org/Portals/42/CCNE/PDF/Procedures.pdf

Davis, W. D., Bellow, A. A., Ramirez, R., & Wilbeck, J. (2020). *Standards of emergency nurse practitioner academic program validation.* https://www.aaenp-natl.org/assets/Standards%20for%20ENP%20Academic%20Program%20Validation%20%285%29.pdf

Davis, W. D., Gibbons Hallman, M., & Wilbeck, J. (2023). Aligning emergency nurse practitioner programs using a national validation process. *Journal for Nurse Practitioners, 19*(7). https://doi.org/10.1016/j.nurpra.2023.104653

International Nursing Association for Clinical Simulation and Learning Standards Committee. (2016). INACSL standards of best practice: Simulation glossary. *Clinical Simulation in Nursing, 12*(S), S39–S47. http://doi.org/10.1016/j.ecns.2016.09.012

National Task Force on Quality Nurse Practitioner Education. (2016). *Standards for quality nurse practitioner education* (5th ed.). https://cdn.ymaws.com/www.nonpf.org/resource/resmgr/docs/evalcriteria2016final.pdf

National Task Force on Quality Nurse Practitioner Education. (2022). *Standards for quality nurse practitioner education* (6th ed.). https://cdn.ymaws.com/www.nonpf.org/resource/resmgr/ntfstandards/ntfs_final.pdf

CHAPTER 7.1

Emergency Nurse Practitioner Certification

Diane Tyler
Lorna Schuman

INTRODUCTION

This section describes the background, purpose, value, and status of specialty certification for emergency nurse practitioners (ENPs). Included is a brief overview of the practice analysis process that is foundational in creating the test specifications and content outline for the American Academy of Nurse Practitioners Certification Board (AANPCB) certification examinations.

BACKGROUND AND NEED

In 2015, the American Academy of Emergency Nurse Practitioners (AAENP) entered into an agreement with AANPCB to develop a specialty certification to recognize eligible family nurse practitioners' (FNPs) expertise in emergency care. Herein is a historical overview of the needs and desire for ENP certification and the rationale for FNP education and certification as requisite to the role.

A key issue was the dissonance between the rise in emergency care visits and an insufficient number of emergency physicians to fill the available positions which continues to be an ongoing concern. With over 141.4 million ED visits in 2014, which represented an 8.9% increase over 2009 ED encounters, the need for emergency and safety net care was evident (Centers for Disease Control and Prevention [CDC], 2013; Rui & Kang, 2014). At the time of initiating the ENP certification program, nurse practitioners (NPs) were providing a significant amount of care in EDs (M. Cook, Vice President, personal communication, February 11, 2018). A report by the Association of American Medical Colleges (AAMC) predicted a shortfall between 42,000 and 121,300 of physicians by the year 2030 in the face of growing demand from an aging population (AAMC, 2018). More recently, when the pandemic was first declared in 2020, there was an initial decrease in ED visits, followed by a large increase in visits (Ghaderi et al., 2021). Although there is an increase in the number of emergency medicine residents, the demand is still expected to outpace the supply, especially in rural and remote areas (Jaret, 2020).

Issues among emergency specialty-care providers, state regulators, and employers involving financial viability and scope of practice also emerged. For example, insurers cited the federal Emergency Medical Treatment and Active Labor Act (EMTALA), which requires all patients be seen regardless of insurance status. The insurance industry lobbied for out-of-network legislation to lower their responsibility of payment for emergency services (American College of Emergency Physicians

[ACEP], 2017). Meanwhile, experienced NPs, particularly FNPs, working in EDs were being required in some states and facilities to obtain acute/critical care academic preparation. However, this challenge to NP scope of practice is not consistent with most patient conditions encountered in EDs. According to the 2010 National Hospital Ambulatory Medical Care Survey (NHAMCS) data, approximately 83% of ED patients were triaged as nonurgent (40%) or as stable needing urgent evaluation with an expected discharge (43%). Similarly, the 2020 NHAMCS data showed that 74.1% of ED patients were discharged and only 14.1% were admitted to the hospital. Thus, the overwhelming majority of ED patients have not needed hospitalization, surgery, or critical care. Furthermore, the CDC (2013) reported age distributions of ED patients as follows: under 15 years old (20%), 15 to 24 years (16%), 25 to 44 years (28%), 45 to 64 (21%), and 65 and older (15%). To meet EMTALA requirements and the needs of patient conditions, emergency care providers must be prepared to treat patients of all ages, which is consistent with FNP educational preparation and scope of practice as the foundation for ENPs. The CDC (2020) data also showed that the ED visit rate for children aged 1 to 15 years was lower than rates for all adult groups, while infant rates were higher compared to other age groups (Cairns et al., 2022).

In addition to ED visit acuity levels and the wide patient age distribution, the geographical need for emergency care services, particularly in rural and underserved areas, was another major consideration for ENP recognition. Approximately 80 million U.S. residents live in health professional shortage areas (AANP, 2020), and NPs, mostly FNPs, accounted for a significant percent (25.2%) of healthcare providers in the rural areas of the United States in 2016 (Barnes et al., 2018; Duquesne University, 2020). Physicians account for only 11% of providers who practice in rural areas (Boyle, 2023). It is also well known that resources for acute, short-term illnesses; minor injuries; and chronic illness management are limited in rural America. Again, providers with a broad scope of care are needed to meet the needs of these communities (AANP, 2022).

Lastly, but no less significant, was the development and refinement of the ENP specialty role in the nursing professional organizations (AAENP [www.aaenp-natl.org]; AANP [www.aanp.org]; and Emergency Nurses Association [www.ena.org]; Hoyt et al., 2018) and growth in the number of emergency care providers among advanced practice nurses. This rapid growth in the ENP specialty, building upon the original ENP competencies (Emergency Nurses Association, 2008), led to the development of the *Scope and Standards of Practice for Emergency Nurse Practitioner Practice* (AAENP, 2016), which have been foundational to the ENP specialty certification program. In 2018, the *Practice Standards for the Emergency Nurse Practitioner Specialty* were developed (AAENP, 2018). These standards define the provision of competent care and foundations of patient care management for the ENP that are reflected within the board certification exam.

PURPOSE

Given this rather complex contextual background and the need for recognition of the specialty knowledge and skills of FNPs working in emergency care, the ENP certification program was created and designed to align with the *Consensus Model for APRN Regulation: Licensure, Accreditation, Certification, and Education* (APRN Consensus Work Group & the National Council of State Boards of Nursing APRN Advisory Committee, 2008) for specialty nursing practice. It was also designed to meet national standards for nursing and healthcare certification program accreditation, which is a requirement for state board of nursing recognition and licensure. Certification for ENPs, as a mechanism for demonstrating the knowledge, skills, and abilities of qualified FNPs who can practice across the life span, provides a legally defensible response to credentialing facilities and agencies, regulators, and insurers for equitable reimbursement of emergency care services. Outcomes data of demonstrating ENP quality patient care are reported elsewhere (Wilbeck et al., 2023).

EMERGENCY NURSE PRACTITIONER PRACTICE ANALYSIS PURPOSE AND PROCESS

The scientific foundations of the ENP certification program consist of national surveys of FNP practice in emergency care. In 2016, the AANPCB conducted the initial practice analysis to develop a new certification program for the advanced practice nursing specialty in emergency care (AANPCB, 2016). The methodology and purpose of a practice analysis are to establish content validity for a certification program and are described elsewhere (Raymond, 2001, 2005). In summary, the process involved identifying and validating the elements of ENP practice; the tasks performed; and the knowledge, skills, and abilities required to perform job tasks (Sackett & Laczo, 2003) of NPs working in emergency care. Ultimately, the practice analysis served to link the exam content outline and test specifications to current emergency specialty practice. The methods of the 2016 practice analysis are described in Tyler et al. (2018). A second practice analysis was conducted in 2021 with updated test specifications that resulted in a slight revision of the practice domains, tasks, and patient conditions (AANPCB, 2021). In addition to providing the basis for constructing and validating a specialty certification examination for ENPs, the findings of the job analyses provide a nationally representative view of current NP emergency practice.

The ENP Scope and Standards (AAENP, 2016), medical, legal, and other current references provide a basis for the development and review of the exam content. Subject matter clinical experts, with diverse practices both geographically and in the types of ED settings, continue to participate in the review and development of each examination.

VALUE OF CERTIFICATION

The value of certification often depends on the profession and includes both intrinsic and extrinsic benefits for professionals. For ENPs, the feeling of pride and a sense of achievement in oneself or one's profession are intrinsic motivators. The certification is evidence of competence, knowledge, and expertise. Certificants may feel more confident when they achieve certification. Salary increases of 5% or more and employability are extrinsic motivators. Other extrinsic motivators include job security, advancement opportunities, enhancement of the public view of the profession, and increased autonomy and/or influence (Roosendaal, 2023).

ENP specialty certification builds upon nationally established standards of NP education and clinical experience (APRN Consensus Work Group & the National Council of State Boards of Nursing APRN Advisory Committee, 2008; National Task Force, 2016, 2022), as well as a commitment to continued education and practice in the role to maintain certification, which is time limited (www.aanpcert.org). The AANPCB certification is accredited by both the Accreditation Board for Specialty Nursing Certification (ABSNC [www.absnc.org]) that accredits nursing certification programs and the National Commission for Certifying Agencies (NCCA [www.credentialingexcellence.org]) that accredits a broad range of professions, including many healthcare certification programs such as nursing, physician assistants, and physicians.

It is important to note that national certification is a higher standard than state licensure. As stated in the *Consensus Model for APRN Regulation*, APRN specialties are not intended to be regulated by state nursing boards. Certification in a specialty area affords NPs an additional method by which they can demonstrate competency through assessment of their specialty knowledge and skills and acknowledgment of their specialty education and clinical expertise.

STATUS OF EMERGENCY NURSE PRACTITIONER CERTIFICATION

Currently, licensure as an ENP is not required for practice; however, some clinical agencies and facilities have recommended ENP certification for employment. The first ENP certification was granted by the American Nurses Credentialing Center (ANCC). A total of 124 NPs across specialties became certified through the portfolio process before it was officially retired in November 2017 (M. Horahan, ANCC Director of Certification, personal communication, October 2017). AANPCB launched the ENP certification by examination in January 2017.

To qualify to take the AANPCB ENP specialty certification examination, the applicant must meet one of the three required eligibility pathways available. One option is the completion of sufficient clinical expertise in advanced emergency care as a nurse practitioner plus specialty continuing education (CE), including emergency-related procedural skills. Another option is the completion of a graduate or postgraduate emergency academic NP program. The third option is the completion of an approved emergency fellowship. As of March 2023, 62% of ENP certificants selected the specialty CE and practice eligibility pathway, 36% qualified via the academic program option, and 2% opted for fellowship eligibility. The eligibility pathways for ENP certification all require additional post-FNP education and clinical experience, which is consistent with other specialty certifications. An active, professional nurse licensure in the United States, U.S. territory, or Canadian province or territory is required to provide assurance to the public that the nurse has met predetermined standards. Due to the life-span scope, applicants must provide verification of current national FNP certification either with AANPCB or ANCC. Information about the eligibility requirements and updated statistics on certification numbers can be found on the AANPCB website at www.aanpcert.org.

CONCLUSION

The ENP certification was developed in response to the public need for competent providers and to address political and economic issues. It was built upon the competencies, unique knowledge, and clinical expertise of practitioners providing emergency care. ENP competencies and practice will continue to evolve, and the ENP certification will reflect the best current evidence for practice.

REFERENCES

American Academy of Emergency Nurse Practitioners. (2016). *Scope and standards for emergency nurse practitioner practice.* https://www.aaenp-natl.org/assets/docs/aaenp_scope_and_standards.pdf
American Academy of Emergency Nurse Practitioners. (2018). *Practice standards for the emergency nurse practitioner specialty.* https://www.aaenp-natl.org/assets/docs/practice_standards_for_the_emergency_nurse_practitioner.pdf
American Academy of Nurse Practitioners Certification Board. (2016). *Report of the 2016 practice analysis of emergency nurse practitioners.* https://www.aanpcert.org/resource/documents/AANPCB%202016%20ENP%20Practice%20Analysis%20Executive%20Summary.pdf
American Academy of Nurse Practitioners Certification Board. (2021). *Practice analysis report: emergency nurse practitioner.* https://www.aanpcert.org/resource/documents/AANPCB%202021%20ENP%20Practice%20Analysis%20Executive%20Summary.pdf

American Association of Nurse Practitioners. (2020). *AANP highlights NP role in providing accessible rural health care during pandemic.* https://www.aanp.org/news-feed/aanp-highlights-np-role-in-providing-accessible-rural-health-care-during-pandemic

American Association of Nurse Practitioners. (2022). *NP fact sheet.* https://www.aanp.org/about/all-abo ut-nps/np-fact-sheet

American College of Emergency Physicians. (2017). *State advocacy issues and resources.* https://www.acep. org/advocacy/stateissues/#sm.0001j34tgo5lhe0rpj5171bg5b29v

APRN Consensus Work Group & the National Council of State Boards of Nursing APRN Advisory Committee. (2008). *Consensus model for APRN regulation: Licensure, accreditation, certification and education.* https://www.aacnnursing.org/Education-resources/APRN-Education/APRN-Consensus-Model

Association of American Medical Colleges. (2018). *The complexities of physician supply and demand: Projections from 2016 to 2030.* https://aamcblack.global.ssl.fastly.net/production/media/filer_public/85/d7/85d7b 689-f417- 4ef0- 97fb-ecc129836829/aamc_2018_workforce_projections_update_april_11_2018.pdf

Barnes, H., Richards, M. R., McHugh, M. D., & Martsolf, G. (2018). Rural and nonrural primary care physician practices increasingly rely on nurse practitioners. *Health Affairs, 37*(6). https://www.healthaffairs .org/doi/10.1377/hlthaff.2017.1158

Boyle, P. (2023, July). *Rural Americans find little escape from climate change.* https://www.aamc.org/news/ru ral-americans-find-little-escape-climate-change#:~:text=Only%2011%25%20of%20physicians%20prac tice,analysis%20by%20the%20Cecil%20G

Cairns, C., Ashman, J. J., & King, J. M. (2022, November). Emergency department visit rates by selected characteristics: United State, 2020. *NCHS Data Brief, 452.*

Centers for Disease Control and Prevention. (2013). *National hospital ambulatory medical care survey factsheet: Emergency department.* https://www.cdc.gov/nchs/data/ahcd/nhamcs_2010_ed_factsheet.pdf

Centers for Disease Control and Prevention. (2020). *National hospital ambulatory medical care survey: 2020 Emergency department summary tables.* https://www.cdc.gov/nchs/data/nhamcs/web_tables/2020-nha mcs-ed-web-tables-508.pdf

Duquesne University. (2020). *Family nurse practitioners meeting health needs in rural areas.* https://onlinenur sing.duq.edu/blog/family-nurse-practitioners-meeting-health-needs-in-rural-areas/

Emergency Nurses Association. (2008). *Competencies for nurse practitioners in emergency care.* https://ww w.ena.org/docs/default-source/education-document-library/enpcompetencies_final.pdf?sfvrsn=f75b 4634_0

Emergency Nurses Association NP Validation Work Team, Hoyt, K. S., Coyne, E. A., Ramirez, E. G., Petard, A. S., Gisness, C., & Gacke-Smith, J. (2010). Nurse practitioner Delphi study: Competencies for practice in emergency care. *Journal of Emergency Nursing, 36,* 439–449. https://doi.org/10.1016/j.jen.2010.05.001

Ghaderi, H., Stowell, J. R., Akhter, M., Norquist, C., Pugsley, P., & Subbian, V. (2021). *Impact of COVID-19 pandemic on emergency department visits: A regional case study of informatics challenges and opportunities,* 496–505. AMIA Annual Symposium Proceedings Archive, 2021

Hoyt, K., Evans, D., Wilbeck, J., Ramirez, E., Agan, D., Tyler, D., & Schumann, L. (2018). Appraisal of the emergency nurse practitioner specialty role. *Journal of the American Association of Nurse Practitioners, 30*(10), 551–559. https://doi.org/10.1097/JXX.0000000000000134

Jaret, P. (2020). *Attracting the next generation of physicians to rural medicine.* https://www.aamc.org/news-in sights/attracting-next-generation-physicians-rural-medicine

National Commission of Certifying Agencies. (2021). *NCCA Standards for the accreditation of certification programs.* https://www.credentialingexcellence.org/Portals/0/NCCA%20Standards%202021%20DRA FT%20REVISIONS_Sept%202021.pdf

National Task Force. (2016). *Criteria for evaluation of nurse practitioner programs* (5th ed.). A report of the national task force on quality nurse practitioner education

National Task Force. (2022). *A report of the national task force on quality nurse practitioner education. Standards for quality nurse practitioner education* (6th ed.). https://www.nonpf.org/page/NTFStandards

Raymond, M. R. (2001). Job analysis and the specification of content for licensure and certification examinations. *Applied Measurement in Education, 14*(4), 369–415.

Raymond, M. R. (2005). An NCME instructional module on developing and administering practice analysis questionnaires. *Educational Measurement: Issues and Practice, 24*(2), 29–42. https://doi.org/10.1111/j. 1745-3992.2005.00009.x

Roosendaal, D. (2023). *The value of certification is more relevant than ever.* https://www.credentialinginsight s.org/Article/the-value-of-certification-is-more-relevant-than-ever-1

Rui, P., & Kang, K. (2014). National hospital ambulatory medical care survey: 2014 emergency department summary tables. https://www.cdc.gov/nchs/data/nhamcs/web_tables/2014_ed_web_tables.pdf

Sackett, P. R., & Laczo, R. M. (2003). Job and work analysis. In W. C. Borman, D. R. Ilgen, R. J. Klimoski, & I. B. Weiner (Eds.), *Handbook of psychology: Industrial and organizational psychology* (Vol. 12, pp. 21–37). John Wiley & Sons.

Tyler, D., Hoyt, K., Evans, D., Schumann, L., Ramirez, E., & Wilbeck, J. (2018). Emergency nurse practitioner practice analysis: Report and implications of the findings. *Journal of the American Association of Nurse Practitioners, 30*(10), 560–569. https://doi.org/10.1097/jxx.0000000000000118

Wilbeck, J., Davis, W., Tyler, D., Schumann, L., & Kapu, A. (2023). Analysis of nurse practitioner practice in U.S. emergency departments: evidence supporting the educational preparation, credentialing, scope of practice & outcomes. *Journal of the American Association of Nurse Practitioners, 35*(6), 373–379. (Submitted to JAANP on 2/20/23)

INDEX